'Wow, what a fantastic book! The straightforward layout is ideal for newcomers, yet detailed enough to complement the more experienced. The instruction methodically guides the practitioner gently through the form, one step at a time. Clear, simple and instantly usable, this work is a valuable addition to any collection.'

– Andrew Austin, ZDL co-founder, world Tai Chi competition medallist

'Laid out in the same format as his previous books, Professor Zhang's book is easy to follow, precise in instruction, and packed with useful detail. The exercises are easy to grasp for beginners with the help of clear directions and excellent photographs, and for the more advanced practitioner, there is a wealth of information.'

– James Drewe, Taiji Ltd, www.taiji.co.uk, author of The Yang Tàijí 24-Step Short Form, Tàijí Jiàn 32-Posture Sword Form, *and* Tai Chi

Dao Yin *for* General Health

by the same author

**Eight Movements to Make the Tendons
and Muscles Supple, Strengthen the Bones
– Shu Jin Zhuang Gu Gong – 1st Form**
Dao Yin Yang Sheng Gong Sequences 3
ISBN 978 1 84819 252 2

**Nourish the Blood, Tonify the Qi to Promote
Longevity, and Calm and Concentrate
the Mind to Regulate the Heart**
Dao Yin Yang Sheng Gong Foundation Sequences 1
ISBN 978 1 84819 072 6

**Thirteen Movements to Stretch the Body and
Make it More Supple, and Guiding and
Harmonising Energy to Regulate the Breath**
Dao Yin Yang Sheng Gong Foundation Sequences 2
ISBN 978 1 84819 071 9

Dao Yin *for* General Health

DAO YIN BAO JIAN GONG – 1ST FORM

导引保健功

PROFESSOR ZHANG GUANGDE

First translation (Chinese-French) by Zhu Mian Sheng
Second translation (French-English) by Mark Atkinson

Commentary by André Perret

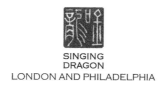

SINGING
DRAGON
LONDON AND PHILADELPHIA

First published in 2016
by Singing Dragon
an imprint of Jessica Kingsley Publishers
73 Collier Street
London N1 9BE, UK
and
400 Market Street, Suite 400
Philadelphia, PA 19106, USA

www.singingdragon.com

Copyright © Zhang Guangde 2016
English translation © Mark Atkinson 2016
Commentary © André Perret 2016

Library of Congress Cataloging in Publication Data
Names: Guangde, Zhang.
Title: Dao yin for general health : dao yin bao jian gong / Professor Zhang
  Guangde.
Other titles: Qi gong geˊneˊral pour preˊserver la santeˊ. English
Description: London ; Philadelphia : Singing Dragon, 2016. | Translation of:
  Qi gong geˊneˊral pour preˊserver la santeˊ.
Identifiers: LCCN 2015042408 | ISBN 9781848193093 (alk. paper)
Subjects: LCSH: Dao yin. | Breathing exercises.
Classification: LCC RA781.85 .G8313 2016 | DDC 613.7/1489--dc23
LC record available at http://lccn.loc.gov/2015042408

British Library Cataloguing in Publication Data
A CIP catalogue record for this book is available from the British Library

ISBN 978 1 84819 309 3
eISBN 978 0 85701 261 6

Printed and bound in Great Britain

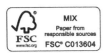

Contents

Professor Zhang Guangde

Born in Tangshan in the province of Hebei, China, in March 1932, Zhang Guangde, Professor at the Beijing University of Physical Education, is one of the greatest masters of Chinese martial arts and has been granted the title of eighth *Duan* in this field.

Professor Zhang is the honorary president of the *Dao Yin* centre of the same university, and former president of the commission of *Dao Yin* of the Association of Higher Education in China.

At the age of 20 he began the practice of martial arts in his home town, and then continued at the Department of Martial Arts at the Beijing University of Physical Education where he completed his studies in 1959. In 1963 he was one of the first generation of graduate research students in this field. He taught martial arts at the university for 45 years and has become one of its most famous graduates.

Professor Zhang has spent more than 40 years creating and developing his own system: *Yang Sheng Tai Ji* and *Dao Yin Yang Sheng*. This system is based on the philosophy of the *I Ching*, as well as the principal theories of Traditional Chinese Medicine such as the meridians, *Yin* and *Yang*, the five elements, *Qi* and blood (*Xue*). The method has shown remarkable effectiveness in maintaining health, as well as for the prevention and treatment of chronic diseases. His work unites six aspects: *I Ching*, medicine, martial arts, art, music, and beauty. Professor Zhang's teaching is imbued with his exceptional personal qualities, and has been received warmly throughout China.

Dao Yin Yang Sheng Gong has gained the National Prize for Technical Progress in Physical Education and a great many other awards.

It forms part of the Chinese national programme for the improvement of the health of the people.

Professor Zhang has written more than 30 books in China, and published scores of articles that have gained many awards in the national congresses of martial arts.

In addition to teaching practitioners who come to China to study *Dao Yin* with him, Professor Zhang has lectured frequently in more than 20 countries including Japan, France, Germany, Australia, Singapore, the United Kingdom, the United States and others, in order to raise awareness of the Chinese culture of wellbeing. Today, millions of people in China and throughout the world practise *Dao Yin Yang Sheng Gong*.

In 2005, he created the International Institute of Dao Yin Yang Sheng Gong (IIDYYSG) in Biarritz, France.

The accompanying video materials can be accessed at: www.jkp.com/voucher using the code ZHANGDAOYIN.

Editorial Preface

*Zhu Mian Sheng, André Perret, Yolande Mano and
Pantxika Iriquin*

For five years, thanks to the commitment of Professor Zhang
Guangde and the pleasure he derives from his teaching, students of
the International Institute of Dao Yin Yang Sheng Gong (IIDYYSG)
gained a high level of development and understanding of this
method. However, the transmission of this knowledge in all its
subtleties has only been possible because of an interpreter with
an outstanding knowledge of Traditional Chinese Medicine and
thought, as well as the techniques of *Dao Yin*: Madam Zhu Mian
Sheng.

The original descriptive text of *Dao Yin Bao Jian Gong*, written
by Professor Zhang Guangde, was initially translated into French
by Madam Zhu Mian Sheng with corrections by the editorial team,
and this English edition is a translation of that work. In doing this
we have tried to reproduce, in the best way possible, the depth and
form of this teaching, both through the choice of the specific terms
used and through the notes and supplementary appendices. In doing
so, we have worked according to certain principles:

1. To translate the original work of Professor Zhang Guangde
   in its entirety as faithfully as possible.

2. To include complementary footnotes, as an aid to developing
   a better understanding of the text.

3. To assume that the reader already understands, albeit perhaps only a little, some basic theory of Traditional Chinese Medicine – *Yin Yang*, *Wu Xing* (the five elements/ movements), *Zhang Fu* (the organs and entrails), and *Jing Luo* (the meridians).

4. To assume that the reader already has some understanding of the principles which form the theoretical and technical base of *Dao Yin Yang Sheng Gong* as explained in *Dao Yin Yang Sheng Gong*, Foundation Sequences 1 and 2 (also published by Singing Dragon), namely: breathing, concentration, stretching, the mobilisation of energy, the preparation common to all sequences, as well as the explanations concerning *Dan Tian* (cinnabar field), *Cai Qi Zhang* (energy collecting palm), *Xiao Zhou Tian* (small celestial cycle), *Que Qiao* (magpie bridge), *Zhan Zhuang* (rooting posture), *Zhong Jian* (central vertical axis) etc.

5. To illustrate the description of the technique with video demonstrations by Zhang Jian in the accompanying video.[1]

6. To improve theoretical understanding by means of a video lecture by Professor Zhang Guangde.

However, it is our view that this sequence merits further technical explanation. For this reason we have included a commentary from Dr André Perret. These comments are based not only on his extensive teaching experience and research, but also and especially on that of Professor Zhang Guangde himself.

The objective of the International Institute is 'to disseminate accurate knowledge of the technique and theory of *Dao Yin Yang Sheng Gong*.' Our hope is that this method does not become distorted through misunderstanding, and that every practitioner may benefit from what is undoubtedly a treasure.

---

1   Available at www.jkp.com/voucher using the code: ZHANGDAOYIN.

PART 1

Eight Movements for General Health

导引保健功

Dao Yin Bao Jian Gong

First form

INTRODUCTION

There are two sequences of *Dao Yin Bao Jian Gong*. They both conform to the global concept of Traditional Chinese Medicine as well as to the theory of 阴阳 *Yin Yang*, with that of 五行 *Wu Xing* (the five elements), 氣 *Qi* (energy), 血 *Xue* (blood) and 经络 *Jing Luo* (the meridians). *Dao Yin Bao Jian Gong* addresses the causes of various common diseases.

This is a sequence of *Dao Yin* in which the movements accord with the system of meridians in order to improve the function of the five organs and six entrails; thus, it has a general action of prevention and treatment for common illnesses.

The experience of more than 30 years of practice shows clearly that this sequence does have favourable effects, which is why it is popular both in China and elsewhere.

The remarkable effectiveness of *Dao Yin Bao Jian Gong* is a consequence of its specific characteristics.

CHARACTERISTICS

1. Combines 形 Xing and 意 Yi, placing the emphasis on Yi

意 *Yi*: idea, intention, concentration, will, thought

形 *Xing*: posture or movement

The practice of the first form of *Dao Yin Bao Jian Gong* requires close coordination between the concentration (*Yi*) and the posture or movement (*Xing*). Having practised and mastered the movements, the emphasis needs to move gradually to the practice of concentration.

In *Dao Yin*, there are different methods depending on the emphasis:

- Focus on concentration is known as 意念导引 *Yi Nian Dao Yin*.

- Focus on posture or movement is known as 姿势导引 *Zi Shi Dao Yin* or 动作导引 *Dong Zuo Dao Yin*.

They have different characteristics and actions in prevention as well as treatment; the one cannot be substituted for the other.

CHARACTERISTICS OF *DAO YIN* FOCUSING ON CONCENTRATION

- While in a state of calm, discover the movement, i.e. through the calmness of concentration, experience the movement within the body.

- Calmness stimulates the circulation of blood throughout the body and promotes the energetic processes of the organs. The meridians, energy and blood are released and regulated, facilitating the circulation of energy between the organs and in the meridians and opening the acupuncture points of the whole body.

CHARACTERISTICS OF *DAO YIN* FOCUSING ON THE MOVEMENT OR POSTURE

- Find calmness within the movement, i.e. through balanced, soft and slow movements, create and experience calmness within the body.

- The movement promotes an energetic equilibrium in the meridians and the viscera, as well as balancing and calming the nervous system.

This is why it is necessary to link the two methods which, when well combined, will help to consolidate correct energy and eliminate perverse energy.

Performing these internal exercises simultaneously strengthens the external, resulting in good health.

If *Dao Yin* through movement produces this important action, one may wonder why, after having mastered the movements, it is then necessary to place the emphasis on the work of concentration.

- The concentration required throughout the sequence is the principal guide of the exercises.

- It is the concentration on certain points that causes the sensation of *Qi* (experiencing energy), which is an essential action of the practice of *Dao Yin*. It could be said that without the action of concentration, a movement cannot be completed in a state of balance.

- Precise concentration is the key to avoiding side effects from the practice, or accidents during the exercises. Anyone practising this sequence, even several times a day, irrespective of time or place, will not experience any side effect or accident as long as the accuracy of the concentration is respected. The principal cause of side effects or accidents is poor concentration, in which tension is used to fix the mind rigidly on a place. In fact this is the opposite of the goal of correct concentration. *Concentration is an integral process in the exercises, but it is not the aim of them.*

- Psychological problems are currently seen as a principal cause of illness. Indeed, nowadays there is a growing view that, with the exception of viruses, psychological and social imbalances are the most important causes of illness. Precise concentration can regulate and rebalance the emotions and the morale, and this is why it is important to link concentration and the movement, placing the emphasis on concentration.

Correct harmonisation of *Yi Nian Dao Yin* (concentration) and *Dong Zuo Dao Yin* (the movement) undoubtedly helps to consolidate correct energy and eliminate perverse energy. Practising internal exercises also consolidates the external, resulting in both physical and psychological good health.

CHARACTERISTICS OF CONCENTRATION IN
DAO YIN BAO JIAN GONG FIRST FORM

- The place of concentration changes according to the posture and the movement. For example:

  ◦ in the first movement 'Regulate the breath', the fourth movement 'The great bird spreads its wings', the fifth movement 'Lift the great stone with power' and the eighth movement 'The ancient sage strokes his beard', the concentration is on 丹田 *Dan Tian*

  ◦ in the second movement 'Push the boat downstream', the sixth movement 'Push the window to look at the moon' and the seventh movement 'Brush the dust into the wind', the concentration is on 劳宫 *Lao Gong* (HP8)

  ◦ in the third movement 'Carry the sun and moon on the shoulders', the concentration is on 命门 *Ming Men* (GV4).

- The place of concentration relates to various disorders.

2. Combines movement and breathing, placing the emphasis on the breathing

动 *Dong*: the movement, the posture

息 *Xi*: breathing; one inhalation and one exhalation equals one breath *Xi*

It is necessary to combine breathing and movement closely, emphasising breathing.

Because *Hu Xi* (respiration) forms part of *Dao Yin*, it is called 呼吸导引 *Hu Xi Dao Yin*.

Both *Dao Yin* through breathing and *Dao Yin* through movement have their own characteristics and action in the prevention and the treatment of disorders and illnesses.

CHARACTERISTICS OF *DAO YIN* THROUGH BREATHING

The regulation of breathing contributes to the clearing of the meridians, the harmonising and balancing of *Yin* and *Yang*, the regulation of energy, the harmonisation of the centre and the regulation of energy and blood.

This is why combining the movement and breathing while emphasising breathing is not only a characteristic of the first form of *Dao Yin Bao Jian Gong* but also a general characteristic of all *Dao Yin Yang Sheng Gong* forms.

It is absolutely essential that practitioners understand and experience these characteristics and continually put them into practice.

3. Relaxes the entire body, experiencing postures and movements that are relaxed and pleasant

The eight movements of this sequence are relaxed, harmonious and supple, free-flowing, light and slow, balanced, pleasurable and natural. They are like the silk worm in the spring that spins its silken thread continuously; like clouds and water flowing without pause.

With practice, this sequence promotes a feeling of expansion of the mind, cheerfulness and purity of spirit. It also releases energy, and the body and mind become light, like that of a sage.

Movements with characteristics such as these help to balance *Yin* and *Yang*, release the meridians, regulate and harmonise energy and blood, invigorate the blood, dissolve stasis, release adhesions, soften the joints, alleviate pain, eliminate swellings, strengthen the tendons, and reinforce the bones in order to fortify the body.

4. For each movement involving rotation, the associated posture involves twisting or curling

This characteristic is found throughout the sequence and indicates that all movements involving the arms and legs will include successive rotations. For example:

- in the first movement 'Regulate the breath', slightly raising the wrists, gently lowering the hands; slowly and gently bending and straightening the legs

- in the third movement 'Carry the sun and moon on the shoulders', the rotation of the trunk to the left and right, the internal and external rotation of the arms, successive rotations of the wrists

- in the sixth movement 'Push the window to look at the moon', the internal rotations of the arms to the left and right describing successive circles, folding and straightening the knees and the ankles, forming 盘根步 *Pan Gen Bu* (twisted posture), coordinating turning the ball of the front foot with bending the ankle of this foot as well as raising the heel of the back foot and pushing the external section of this foot, and also the turning of the lumbar region and the extending the chest

- in the seventh movement 'Brush the dust into the wind', the successive rotation of the arms; the series of folding and pushing the elbows, extending the hands to 'brush the dust'.

All these movements function as if the fingers are being used as acupuncture needles to:

- release the energetic mechanism of the whole body

- regulate and harmonise *Yin* and *Yang*

- reinforce the functions of the internal organs

- regulate the nervous system

- increase the functions of the heart and lung, reduce cholesterol, and regulate the blood pressure.

5. Contracts and relaxes 谷道 Gu Dao (the anus), closely linking this action with breathing[2]

When inhaling, closely coordinate the movements of the anal and perineal muscles with the breathing; this coordination is required in each movement.

6. The movements are soft, slow, balanced, harmonious, successive and continuous

In this sequence, it is necessary to pay attention to the four 'principles' and the four 'prohibitions'.

FOUR PRINCIPLES

- the movements should be slow

- they should be soft and harmonious

- they should be successive, i.e. without pause

- they should be dynamic throughout.

---

2   In spite of the pressure in the lower abdomen induced by the contraction of the perineum, the breathing remains abdominal. This is fully described in *Dao Yin Yang Sheng Gong, Foundation Sequences 2*, Singing Dragon.

FOUR PROHIBITIONS

- stiffness or hardness
- slackness
- absence of 'roundedness'
- abruptness or lack of continuity.

The four principles and the four prohibitions are related. We use the one to avoid the others. Slowness helps softness; softness helps vitality; vitality helps continuity; continuity helps softness.

If the four principles are well combined and the four prohibitions avoided, the result is a carefree, peaceful and serene state of mind, with a feeling of lightness and flexibility in the body, purity of spirit and tranquillity of energy, supported by a beautiful and balanced posture.

In practice, if one always respects this association of the four principles with the four prohibitions, one can:

- release and regulate the meridians
- harmonise *Qi* (energy) and *Xue* (blood) and thus free the energetic mechanism of the five organs
- reinforce energy to nourish the blood
- dissolve blockages and stasis, in order to strengthen the body and prevent and treat chronic diseases.

TITLES OF THE EIGHT MOVEMENTS

First movement: Regulate the breath

调息吐纳 *Tiao Xi Tu Na*

Second movement: Push the boat downstream

顺水推舟 *Shun Shui Tui Zhou*

Third movement: Carry the sun and moon on the shoulders

肩担日月 *Jian Dan Ri Yue*

Fourth movement: The great bird spreads its wings

鹏鸟展翅 *Peng Niao Zhan Chi*

Fifth movement: Lift the great stone with power

力搬磐石 *Li Ban Pan Shi*

Sixth movement: Push the window to look at the moon

推窗望月 *Tui Chang Wang Yue*

Seventh movement: Brush the dust into the wind

迎风掸尘 *Ying Feng Dan Chen*

Eighth movement: The ancient sage strokes his beard

老翁拂髯 *Lao Weng Fu Ran*

PREPARATION

Movement

1. Stand with feet together, body upright, balanced.

2. Look ahead.

3. The eyes may be lightly closed.

4. The tip of the tongue touches the palate, the teeth are lightly touching.

5. Bring the hands to the surface of *Dan Tian*, the left hand in contact with this zone for both men and women.

6. Silently recite the poem of preparation.

   It is night, everything is silent.
   Dismiss the 10,000 problems of life.
   Concentrate the mind on Dan Tian
   And keep well closed the seven openings of the face.
   Breathe deeply, slowly, softly
   And make the 'magpie bridge'.
   The body is light like a swallow in the springtime
   Which swoops and flies towards the distant clouds.

7. At the end of the preparation, lower the arms alongside the body.

FIRST MOVEMENT: REGULATE THE BREATH

调 息 吐 纳 *Tiao Xi Tu Na*

Meaning of the title

The characters 调 息 吐 纳 *Tiao Xi Tu Na* mean to regulate the respiration.

In ancient China, it was a method of 养生 *Yang Sheng*, that is to say, a means of nourishing vitality. It was used to expel the maximum amount of impure energy through the mouth, then to assimilate pure energy through the nose. In the book *Zhuang Zi*, it is referred to as *Tu Gu Na Xin*: to spit out the old and swallow the new.

Ji Kang, a Taoist master of the time, explained in his book *Studies of Yang Sheng*, 'Through respiration (*Tu Na*), energy is absorbed to nourish vitality.' Taoist practices accord with this theory which proposes that by *Tu Na* it is possible to assimilate *Sheng Qi* (dynamic energy) and expel *Si Qi* (dead energy) and thus attain longevity.

MOVEMENT

1. Inhaling, contract 谷道 *Gu Dao* (the anus) and tighten the perineum. Place the bodyweight onto the right foot, bending the right knee slightly. Step to the left, feet slightly more than shoulder width apart. Straighten the legs, equalising the bodyweight between the feet. Simultaneously, leading with the backs of the wrists, raise the arms forward, palms facing the floor, to shoulder height and shoulder width. Naturally extend the arms, elbows downward. Look ahead.

2. Exhaling, relax *Gu Dao* and the perineum, and bend the knees slightly. At the same time, lower the elbows, bend the wrists slightly and push the hands forward at the height of the navel, palms downward, fingers pointing forward. Look ahead.

3. Inhaling, contract *Gu Dao* and tighten the perineum. Bend the knees. Simultaneously, leading with the heel of the hand, push the hands forward. Then straighten the knees, and, leading with the point of the wrist, raise the hands to shoulder height, keeping them shoulder width apart. Look ahead.

Elements 4 and 6 are the same as 2, 5 and 7 the same as 3.

8. Exhaling, relax *Gu Dao* and the perineum. Move the bodyweight onto the right foot; bring the left foot next to the right foot. Gradually straighten the legs. At the same time, lower the arms alongside the body. Look ahead.

REPETITIONS

Perform elements 1–8 twice.

Begin the second round of 8 by stepping out with the right foot.

KEY POINTS

- In order to advance and raise the hands, it is necessary to lower the shoulders and slightly bend the elbows, and not push the belly out.

- When bending the knees, draw in the buttocks and lower the pelvis; do not lean forward or backward.

- Point of concentration: 丹田 *Dan Tian* or 劳宫 *Lao Gong* (HP8).

SECOND MOVEMENT: PUSH THE BOAT DOWNSTREAM

顺 水 推 舟 *Shun Shui Tui Zhou*

Meaning of the title

Shun Shui Tui Zhou means to act so that you benefit from the circumstances. Here the title is used to indicate to practitioners that they should relax their minds and calm their emotions while making their movements continuous, without pausing, like a boat that moves along with a current.

MOVEMENT

1. Inhaling, contract *Gu Dao* (the anus) and tighten the perineum. Turn the body to the left, 45°, then move the bodyweight onto the right foot, bending the right knee. Step obliquely forward with the left foot, placing the heel on the ground in order to form 左虚步 *Zuo Xu Bu* (the 'empty' step). At the same time, straighten the arms naturally. Leading with the back of the wrist, raise the hands obliquely forward and to shoulder height. Then, following a slight rotation of the trunk to the right, bend and lower the elbows, bringing the hands in front of the shoulders, palms forward. Look forward to the left diagonal.

2. Exhaling, relax *Gu Dao* and the perineum; lower the bodyweight and move it onto the left foot to form 左弓步 *Zuo Gong Bu* (the 'bow' step). At the same time, lower the hands to waist level. Then, bend the wrists, bringing the fingers upward. Straighten the arms naturally, dropping the elbows, as if pushing a boat in the direction of the current. Experience a feeling of being at ease, of flexibility. Look ahead.

3. Inhaling, contract *Gu Dao* and tighten the perineum. Move
    the bodyweight onto the right foot, bending the right knee
    slightly, straightening the left leg. Raise the toes of the left
    foot to form *Zuo Xu Bu*. At the same time, relax the wrists,
    directing the palms downwards. Following a slight rotation
    of the trunk to the right, then to the left, drop the elbows.
    The hands then describe an upward circle, bringing them in
    front of the chest, palms forward and fingers upward. Look
    forward.

Element 4 is the same as 2, element 5 the same as 3, element 6 the
same as 2.

7. Inhaling, contract *Du Dao* and tighten the perineum. Move
    the bodyweight onto the right foot, bending the right knee
    and straightening the left leg. Raise the toes of the left foot
    to form *Zuo Xu Bu*; straighten the arms, palms naturally
    downward. Then, turn the body to face forward again.
    Led by the body movement, the hands describe a circle to
    the right, parallel to the ground and at shoulder height;
    straighten the arms, palms naturally downward. Look ahead.

8. Exhaling, relax *Du Dao*, the perineum. Bring the left foot
    back beside the right foot, and then straighten the legs
    gradually, at the same time lowering the arms alongside the
    body. Look ahead.

Repetitions

Perform elements 1–8 twice.

Perform the second series of 8 beginning by stepping out on
the right foot.

Key points

- When forming 虚步 *Zuo Xu Bu*, relax the lumbar region and draw in the buttocks. Do not lean the trunk backward or forward.

- When forming 左弓步 *Zuo Gong Bu*, do not push the buttocks out. Keep the lumbar region relaxed, lower the buttocks and place the back heel firmly on the ground.

- Point of concentration: 劳宫 *Lao Gong* (HP8).

THIRD MOVEMENT: CARRY THE SUN AND MOON ON THE SHOULDERS

肩担日月 *Jian Dan Ri Yue*

Meaning of the title

This title comes from a story. In ancient times a young, well-read man took part in the state examinations, having already been successful at the provincial and capital level. The exam remaining was to be taken in front of the emperor. The emperor had read his file and was impressed with the young man's results, but he did not know anything about his family situation or his ability to express himself. At the moment of the examination, the emperor did not ask him a question about the economy or the management of a state, but instead asked him only this: 'What work is done by your grandparents and your parents?'

The young man was anxious when he heard this because his grandfather manufactured alcohol and his grandmother carded cotton; his father sold tofu in the street that his mother made in their home. He thought that if he simply said that to the emperor, he would lose the contest, but at the same time he could not lie to the emperor.

Relying on his sharp wits and keen mind, he quietly answered the emperor by saying: 'Thanks to your protection, my grandfather cares for the jade pots which open the eye of Heaven and Earth; my grandmother handles a golden hammer which can awake the heart of the emperor; my mother turns *Qian Kun*[3] in our home, and my father carries the sun and moon outside on his shoulders.'

The emperor was very satisfied with this answer and the young man gained his examination with the highest mark.

---

3   *Qian* is one of the eight classical trigrams that signify the sky/heaven; *Kun* is one of the eight classical trigrams that signify the earth.

MOVEMENT

1. Inhaling, contract *Gu Dao* (the anus) and tighten the perineum. Turn the body 90° to the left. Following an internal rotation of the arms, describe a circle to raise the hands to shoulder height, palms upward. Then, following an external rotation of the arms, turn the palms upward, then bend and drop the elbows to form an angle of 90° between the arms and the body and an angle of 120° between the forearm and the arm, palms upward, fingers directed sideways. Look at the left hand. This posture is as if the front hand carries the sun and the back hand carries the moon. It suggests light, the brightness of the sun and the moon heating the five organs, the six entrails and the heart.

2. Exhaling, relax the *Gu Dao*, the perineum. Turn the body to the front again, then, following the rotation of the trunk, with an internal rotation of the arms and wrists, describe a circle with the hands to bring the palms upward, fingers pointing backward. Look at the left hand. Without pausing, lower the hands forward, then bring the arms alongside the body. Look ahead.

Elements 3, 5 and 7 are the same as 1, elements 4, 6 and 8 the same as 2.

Repetitions

Perform elements 1–8 twice.

At the end of the second series of 8, bring the hands in front of the pelvis, palms upward, fingers pointing toward each other. Keep a distance of approximately 10cm between the tips of the fingers and between the hands and the stomach. Look ahead.

Key points

- In this movement, relax the entire body, open the chest, release the shoulders and drop the elbows. The hands are above the shoulders, the elbows below the shoulders.

- Rotate the body as much as possible while remaining upright. Do not lean to the left or right, forward or backward.

- Point of concentration: 命门 *Ming Men* (GV4).

FOURTH MOVEMENT: THE GREAT BIRD SPREADS ITS WINGS

鹏鸟展翅 *Peng Niao Zhan Chi*

Meaning of the title

In Chinese mythology, *Peng* was an immense bird that had transformed from an equally enormous fish named *Kun*. In its incarnation as a bird it could accomplish a flight of 10,000 *Li* (5,000 km) with a single sweep of its wings. In China, the title of this exercise is used as a phrase to indicate that someone has a brilliant future, one that it is full of promise.

MOVEMENT

1. Inhaling, contract *Gu Dao* (the anus) and tighten the perineum. Move the bodyweight onto the right foot, bending the right knee slightly. Open the left foot sideways, to a distance between the feet a little more than shoulder width. Then, equalise the bodyweight between the feet and gradually straighten the knees. At the same time, open the hands sideways and upward in a circle until they are above the head. The arms form a circle, palms upward, fingers facing inward. This posture imitates a bird spreading its wings. Look ahead.

2. Exhaling, relax *Gu Dao* and the perineum. Move the bodyweight onto the right foot, slightly bending the right knee. Then, bring the left foot next to the right and gradually straighten the legs. At the same time, lower the arms sideways until they return in front of the belly to their starting position (as described above). This posture imitates a bird closing its wings. Look ahead.

Elements 3 and 4 are the same as 1 and 2, but beginning by stepping to the right.

5. Inhaling, contract *Gu Dao*, and tighten the perineum. Lower the bodyweight onto the right foot, slightly bending the right knee. Advance the left foot, then place the heel on the floor, raising the toes of this foot to form 左虚步 *Zuo Xu Bu* (the 'empty' step). Then, progressively move the bodyweight onto the left foot, straightening both legs, and raising the right heel. At the same time, the hands describe an arc of a circle forward and upward until they arrive above the head, the palms turning upward, the arms forming a circle. Look ahead.

6. Exhaling, relax *Gu Dao* and the perineum. Move the bodyweight onto the right foot, lowering the heel to the ground, slightly bending the right knee. Simultaneously, straighten the left leg, raising the toes. Then bring the left foot beside the right foot, gradually straightening the legs. At the same time, lower the hands by describing an arc of a circle forward and downward until they arrive in front of the pelvis; the arms form a circle, palms upward. Look ahead.

Elements 7 and 8 are the same as 5 and 6, but beginning by advancing the right foot.

Repetitions

Repeat elements 1–8 twice.

Key points

- Open the chest and relax the whole body when raising the hands above the head. Lift the heel of the back foot as much as possible. When returning the hands in front of the belly, close the chest slightly in order to draw energy down. Pay attention to coordinating the movements of the upper and lower limbs.

- Point of concentration: 丹田 *Dan Tian.*

FIFTH MOVEMENT: LIFT THE GREAT STONE WITH POWER

力搬磐石 *Li Ban Pan Shi*

Meaning of the title

Pan Shi are thick, heavy stones, such as millstones. The title is used here to suggest the stability and solidity of the foot, and to indicate that the foot can support heavy loads.

In China, as the life of stones is much longer than that of animals or plants, it is common to refer to 寿石 *Shou Shi* as stones of longevity. This is why longevity stones with beautiful images of the Mother of the West are often found in Chinese paintings as wishes for long life. Such images wish for the recipient a life as rich and full of happiness as the Mother of the West, and a longevity as solid as that of Mount Nanshan.

According to legend, longevity stones, especially the stones of the Taishan mountain (revered by Taoists), can drive out evil spirits. Monsters of any kind are afraid of these stones and avoid them.

MOVEMENT

1. Inhaling, contract *Gu Dao* (the anus) and tighten the perineum. Move the bodyweight onto the right foot, slightly bending the right knee. Step sideways with the left foot to a distance about equal to three times the length of the foot, then equalise the bodyweight between the feet, gradually straightening the legs. At the same time, raise the hands to chest height, palms upward, fingers facing each other. Keep the hands within the field of vision. Without pausing, and following an internal rotation of the arms, describe a circle with the hands that pass in front of the face, then to each side. Then, gradually straighten the arms, palms obliquely forward. Look ahead.

2. Exhaling, relax *Gu Dao* and the perineum. Slowly bend the legs to form *Ma Bu* (horseriding posture). Following an internal rotation of the forearms, direct the palms downwards, fingers pointing sideways. Describe a circle downward and inward with the hands until they are a little lower than the knees, palms upward. The arms form a circle with palms upward, fingers facing inward, separated by approximately 10cm. This posture represents 'taking hold of the great stone'. The trunk and the head should not be inclined in any direction. Keep the hands within the field of vision.

3. Inhaling, contract *Gu Dao* and tighten the perineum. Straighten the legs. At the same time, raise the hands to chest height and, following an internal rotation of the arms, pass the hands in front of the face, then circle them to each side. Straighten the arms, palms obliquely outward. Look ahead.

Elements 4 and 6 are the same as 2, elements 5 and 7 the same as 3.

8. Exhaling, relax *Gu Dao* and the perineum. Move the bodyweight onto the right foot, bending the right knee. Then, bring the left foot back beside the right and gradually straighten the legs. At the same time, bring the hands in front of the belly, palms upward, fingers facing each other, approximately 10cm apart and 10cm in front of the body. Look ahead.

Repetitions

Perform the series of elements 1–8 twice – once stepping to the left, once stepping to the right.

At the end of the second element 8, bring the right foot back beside the left, then gradually straighten the legs, lowering the hands alongside the body. Look ahead.

Key points

- When lowering the body to form *Ma Bu*, do not lean the upper body or lower the head. When raising the body, push *Bai Hui* (GV20) upward and drop the shoulders.

- Use the mind and not physical force to raise the hands. The 'great stone' should be raised by intention and concentration.

- Point of concentration: 丹田 *Dan Tian*.

SIXTH MOVEMENT: PUSH THE WINDOW TO LOOK AT THE MOON

推窗望月 *Tui Chang Wang Yue*

Meaning of the title

In ancient times, the moon was also known as *Tai Yin*, and it orbited the earth, as it does now.

According to Chinese legend, a beautiful lady called Chang Ge lived on the moon. This came about because her husband, Hou Yi, had been given a drug by Xi Wang Mu, mother of the celestial emperor, which would enable him to become immortal. However, unbeknown to Hou Yi, Chang Ge took this drug herself, and became so light that she flew away to the Palace of the Moon, where she had to remain.

This title indicates that we must be in harmony with our natural environment in order to find the unity of Heaven and mankind.

MOVEMENT

1. Inhaling, contract *Gu Dao* (the anus) and tighten the perineum. Turn the body slightly to the left. At the same time, following an internal rotation of the right arm, turn the right palm forward; raise this arm by describing a circle left and upward, bending the arm slightly to bring the hand in front of the left shoulder. Simultaneously, following an internal rotation of the left arm, push the hand toward the left. When the hand arrives slightly above the hip, make an external rotation of the left arm and continue to raise it to the left; naturally straighten the arm, palm forward. Look at the left hand.

2. Exhaling, relax *Gu Dao*, the perineum. Move the bodyweight onto the right foot, slightly bending the right knee. Turn the body slightly to the right, and take a large step sideways

with the left foot, directing the toes inward. At the same time, continue the movements of the arms, passing the hands in front of the face, then describing a circle toward the right, naturally straightening the right arm, cocking the right wrist to direct the fingers upward. The left hand comes inside the right elbow, palm towards the right, fingers upward. Look at the right hand.

3. Inhaling, contract *Gu Dao* and tighten the perineum. Using the ball of the left foot as a pivot, turn the left heel inward to bring the toes forward. Then, move the bodyweight onto the left foot, slightly bending the left knee. Move the right foot behind the left foot, place it on the ground and slightly bend the right knee. At the same time, the hands describe a circle beginning from the right side toward the left side of the trunk; the left arm arrives in front of the chest on the left, the right arm on the right side of the body. Look at the right hand.

4. Exhaling, relax *Gu Dao* and the perineum. Bend the knees to form 盘根步 *Pan Gen Bu* (twisted roots posture).[4] At the same time, continue to describe a circle with the hands towards the left, pushing them toward the left side. The left hand is slightly higher than the shoulder, palm toward the left, fingers forward; naturally straighten the left arm. Slightly bend the right arm, fingers forward, as if 'pushing the window to look at the moon'. Look through and beyond the left 虎口 *Hu Kou* (tiger's mouth)[5] into the distance.

5. Inhaling, contract *Gu Dao*, and tighten the perineum. Remaining in *Pan Gen Bu*, push the hands first downward, then toward the left in a circle until they arrive in front

---

4   When the foot has crossed behind, the aim is to bend the knees and lower the pelvis to sit between the feet, legs crossed. In practice, lower the body according to individual capabilities.

5   The space between the thumb and index finger.

of the trunk, then move all the bodyweight onto the left foot; bring the right foot back beside the left foot, then gradually straighten the legs. At the same time, following an internal rotation of the left arm, direct the palm forward, raise it upward and to the right, bringing the left hand in front of the right shoulder, slightly bending the left arm. Simultaneously, following an internal then an external rotation of the right arm, raise that arm upward and to the right to shoulder height; naturally straighten the arm, palm forward. Look at the right hand.

6. Exhaling, relax *Gu Dao* and the perineum. Move the bodyweight onto the left foot, slightly bend the left knee; turn the upper body slightly to the left, and take a large step to the right with the right foot, toes pointing inward. At the same time, continue the movements of the arms upward, the hands describing a circle and passing in front of the face, toward the right side of the body. Bring the right hand inside the left elbow, palm toward the left, fingers upward. Straighten the left arm naturally, folding the wrist and directing the fingers upward. Look at the left hand.

7. Inhaling, contract *Gu Dao* and tighten the perineum. Using the ball of the right foot as a pivot, turn the heel inward to bring the toes forward. Then, move the bodyweight onto the right foot, and slightly bend the right knee. Bring the left foot behind the right foot, and place it on the ground to the right, bending the left knee. At the same time, following an internal rotation of the right arm and a slight external rotation of the left arm, the hands pass from the left of the body toward the right. They describe a circle, bringing the right arm in front of the chest, on the left; the left arm remains on the left side. Look at the left hand.

8. Exhaling, relax *Gu Dao* and the perineum. Bend the legs to form *Pan Gen Bu*; at the same time, continue to describe a circle with the hands toward the right and push the hands toward the right side, palms to the right, fingers pointing forward. Straighten the right arm; slightly bend the left arm, fingers forward as if 'pushing the window to look at the moon'. Look through and beyond the right *Hu Kou* into the distance.

Repetitions

Perform elements 1–8 twice.

In the second round, of element, continue the movement to include *Pan Gen Bu*, 'pushing the window'.

Then, on the second round of element 8, from *Pan Gen Bu*, raise the body, bending the knees slightly.

At the same time, first lower the hands, palms downward to bring them in front of the thighs; then raise the arms to shoulder level. Bring the left foot back beside the right foot, gradually straighten the legs, lower the arms alongside the body. Look ahead.

Key points

- To ensure the circularity of the movements and the rotation of the arms, it is necessary to relax the body completely and to make these movements with flexibility; it is essential to coordinate the hand movements with *Pan Gen Bu*.

- When in *Pan Gen Bu*, keep the body upright; direct the point of the front foot toward the outside, legs well intertwined. The insides of the thighs press strongly together and massage each other.

- Point of concentration: 劳宫 *Lao Gong* (HP8).

SEVENTH MOVEMENT: BRUSH THE DUST INTO THE WIND

迎风撣尘 *Ying Feng Dan Chen*

Meaning of the title

Ying Feng Dan Chen indicates not only getting rid of dust from the exterior of the body, but also driving out unwanted thoughts, thus purifying the mind, enabling us to work in a holistic way, internally at the level of *Jing* (the spirit), and externally at the level of *Xing* (the posture and movement).

MOVEMENT

1. Inhaling, contract *Gu Dao* (the anus) and tighten the perineum. Turn the upper body 45° to the left. At the same time, following an internal rotation of the arms, raise the hands left and right sideways, describing a circle so that they arrive slightly lower than the shoulders, the arms naturally extended, palms backward. Look ahead. Without pausing, turn the body slightly to the right. At the same time, following an external rotation of the arms, direct the palms upward, keeping the arms naturally extended. Then, following a slight rotation of the upper body towards the left, move the bodyweight onto the right foot, slightly bending the right knee, and advancing the left foot to form left 左虚步 *Zuo Xu Bu* (the 'empty' step). At the same time, continue the external rotation of the arms and describe a circle upward, forward, then inward (bending the elbows), bringing the backs of the little fingers to the chest, fingers pointing upward. Look toward the left.

2. Exhaling, relax *Gu Dao* and the perineum. Slowly lower the bodyweight, then move it onto the front foot, forming 左弓步 *Zuo Gong Bu* (the 'bow' step). At the same time, slide the

hands down the chest and outward toward the hips. Then, following an internal rotation of the arms, describe a large circle bringing the hands in front of the body, arms naturally extended, palms turned outward. This movement represents 'brushing the dust from the body'. Look ahead to the left.

3. Inhaling, contract *Gu Dao* and tighten the perineum. Move the bodyweight onto the right foot, bend the right knee and straighten the left leg, raising the toes of the left foot to form *Zuo Xu Bu*. Simultaneously, turn the upper body slightly to the right; following an external rotation of the arms, the hands describe a circle in front of the chest and the fingers once again touch each side of the chest, fingers upward. Look ahead to the left.

Elements 4 and 6 are the same as 2, elements 5 and 7 the same as 3.

8. Exhaling, relax *Gu Dao* and the perineum. Turn the upper body forward to form *Zuo Xu Bu*. At the same time, with an internal then an external rotation of the arms, push the hands sideways, palms upward. Look ahead.[6] Without pausing, return the left foot next to the right foot; gradually straighten the legs. Then, pass the hands in front of the face, describing a circle and pushing the hands downward toward the belly, palms downward, fingers facing inward; the arms form a circle. Look ahead.

Repetitions

Perform elements 1–8 twice.

The second time, at the end of element 8, lower the arms alongside the body.

---

6   In recent seminars, Professor Zhang Guangde has altered this description slightly. This stage of the movement, arms spread, palms upward, corresponds to the end of element 7, i.e. the end of the inhalation. The exhalation of element 8 begins with closing the feet and lowering the hands. The main text describes the original movement.

Key points

- Before advancing or returning the foot, first stabilise the bodyweight.

- Make the arm rotations as full as possible. Coordinate the movements of the upper and lower limbs.

- Place of concentration: 劳宫 *Lao Gong* (HP8).

EIGHTH MOVEMENT: THE ANCIENT SAGE STROKES HIS BEARD

老翁拂髯 *Lao Weng Fu Ran*

Meaning of the title

When Chinese people exceed the age of 70 and their hair or beards become white, they are referred to as *Lao Weng*.

In this movement, visualise an old person with a long beard. Smoothing the beard indicates someone who is very wise.

MOVEMENT

1. Inhaling, contract *Gu Dao* (the anus) and tighten the perineum. Move the bodyweight onto the right foot, slightly bending the right knee, and raising the left heel. At the same time, following an internal rotation of the arms, direct the palms downward, fingers forward. Look to the left. Without pausing, step sideways to the left with the left foot to a distance slightly more than the width of the shoulders, toes forward. At the same time, following an internal rotation of the arms, lift the hands to each side of the body, naturally extending the arms, palms backward.[7] Look at the left hand. Without stopping, move the bodyweight onto the left foot, bending the left knee and straightening the right leg. At the same time, following an external rotation of the arms,[8] turn the palms upward, slightly bending the arms. Look at the left hand.

2. Exhaling, relax *Gu Dao* and the perineum. Bring the right foot next to the left foot, gradually straightening the legs.

---

7 In his teaching, Professor Zhang Guangde emphasises the importance of maximum rotation. The maximum internal rotation of the palms therefore brings the palms upward.

8 The maximum rotation of the wrists.

At the same time, describing a circle, bring the hands upward in front of the face, then 'grasp the beard' using 虎 口 *Hu Kou* (tiger's mouth) and push the hands forward and downward in front of the chest; the arms form a circle, palms downward, *Hu Kou* forward. Look ahead.

Elements 3, 5 and 7 are the same as 1, elements 4, 6 and 8 the same as 2.

Repetitions

Perform elements 1–8 twice.

During the second sequence of 1–8, make the same arm movements, but do not move the legs.

On the last movement, lower the arms alongside the body. Look ahead.

Key points

- Relax the entire body; balance and coordinate the movements of the upper and lower limbs.

- When the hands 'take hold of the beard' and push downward, first push the point 百会 *Bai Hui* (GV20) upward to portray an expression of wisdom.

- After finishing the sequence, remain calm for a few moments to gain the most benefit from the practice. It is not helpful to leave the practice place immediately.

- Place of concentration: 丹田 *Dan Tian*.

CLOSING

1. Cross the hands and place them on the surface of 丹田 *Dan Tian*, the left hand touching the body for men, the right hand for women.

2. Remain for a few moments, then lower the arms alongside the body. Look ahead.

POINTS USED

百会 *Bai Hui (GV20)*
On the top of the head, where the midline of the skull crosses a line connecting the tops of the ears.

劳宫 *Lao Gong (HP8)*
In the palm of the hand, between the 2nd and 3rd metacarpal, where the tip of the middle finger touches when the fist is closed.

命门 *Ming Men (GV4)*
In the lumbar region on the posterior midline in a depression, below the spinous process of the 2nd lumbar vertebra (L2).

丹田 *Dan Tian (the cinnabar field)*
This area includes the points *Shen Que* (CV8), in the centre of the navel, *Qi Hai* (CV6), 1.5 cun below the navel, *Guan Yuan* (CV4), 3 cun below the navel and *Tian Shu* (St25), 2 cun either side of *Shen Que* (CV8) and the zone of *Hu Kou*.

虎口 *Hu Kou*
The tiger's mouth, the area between the thumb and index finger.

PHOTOGRAPHS

Preparation

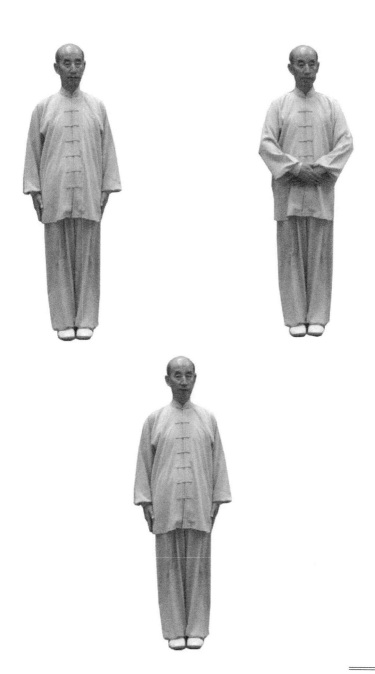

First movement: Regulate the breath

调息吐纳 *Tiao Xi Tu Na*

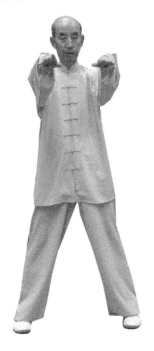

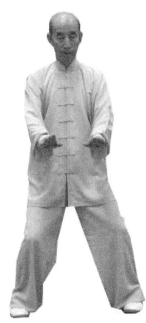

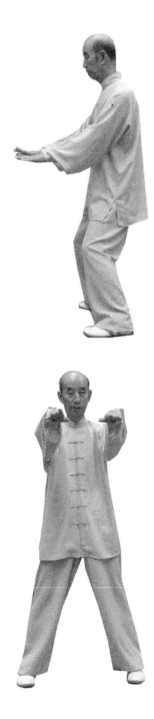

Second movement: Push the boat downstream

順 水 推 舟 *Shun Shui Tui Zhou*

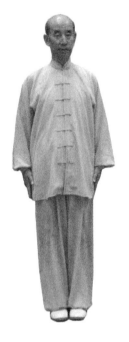

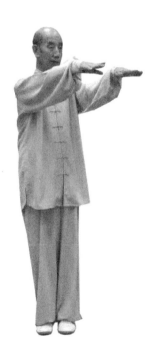

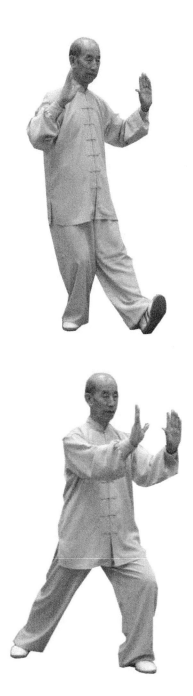

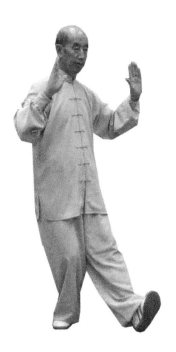

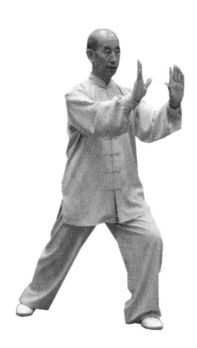

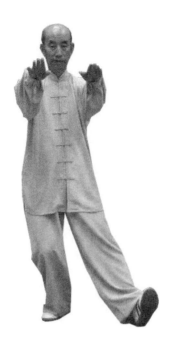

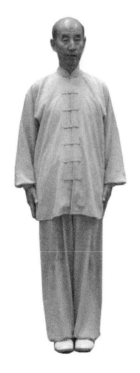

Third movement: Carry the sun and moon on the shoulders

肩担日月 *Jian Dan Ri Yue*

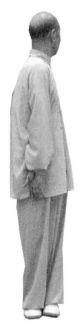

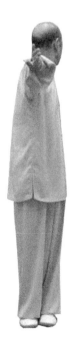

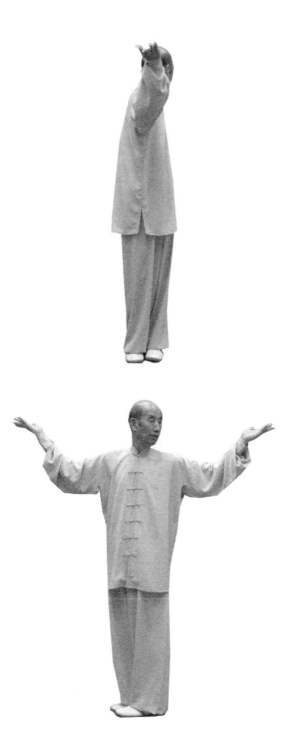

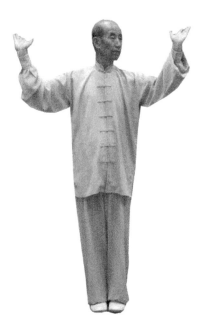

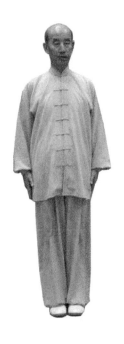

Fourth movement: The great bird spreads its wings

鹏鸟展翅 *Peng Niao Zhao Chi*

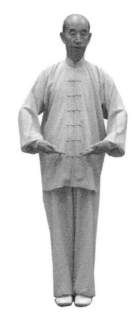

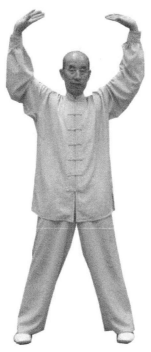

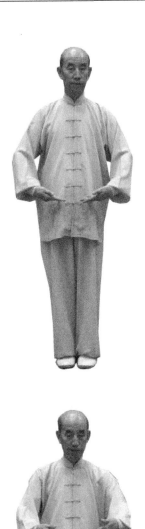

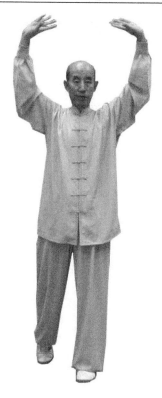

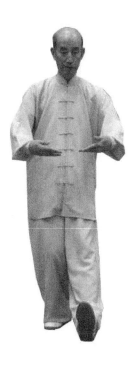

Fifth movement: Lift the great stone with power

力搬磐石 *Li Ban Pan Shi*

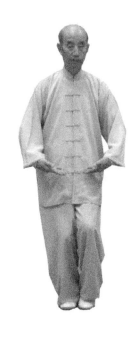

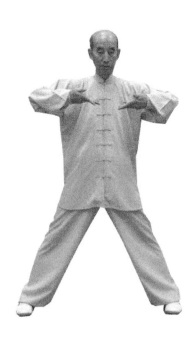

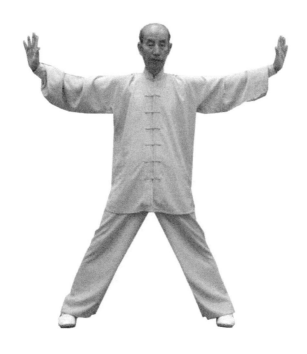

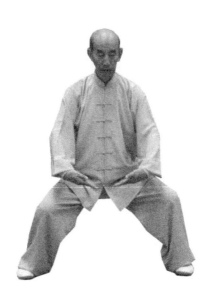

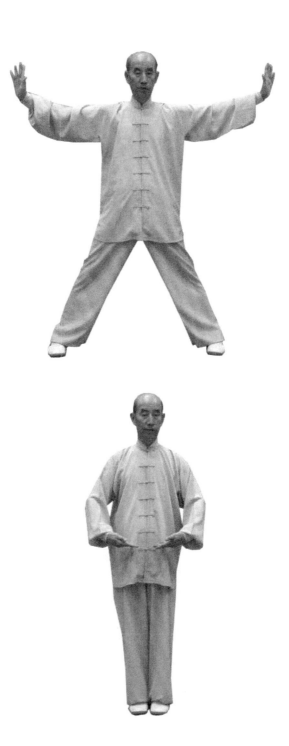

Sixth movement: Push the window to look at the moon

推窗望月 *Tui Chang Wang Yue*

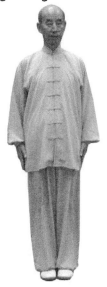

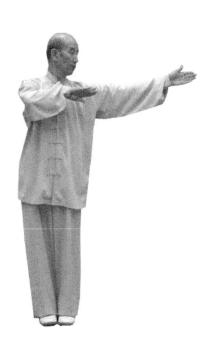

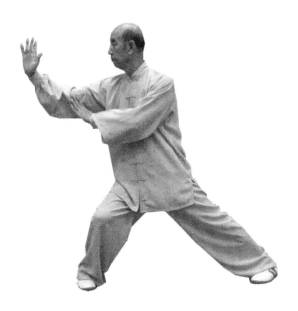

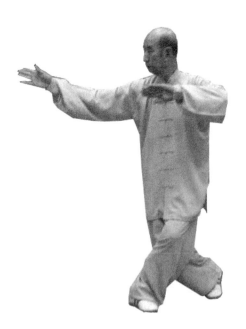

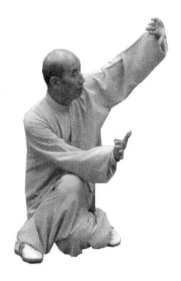

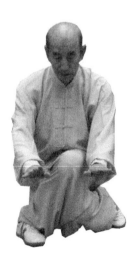

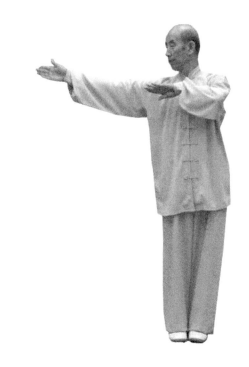

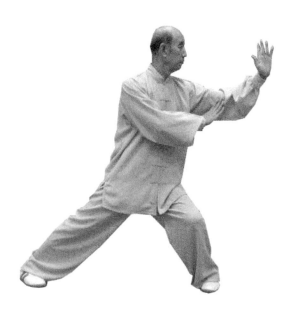

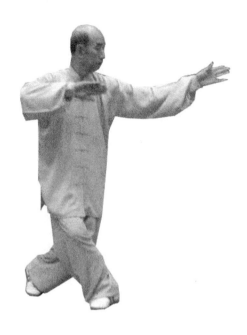

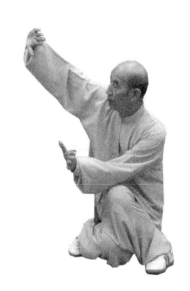

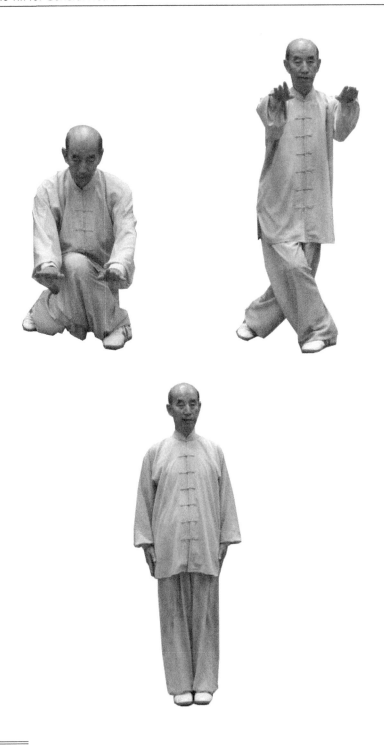

Seventh movement: Brush the dust into the wind

迎风掸尘 *Ying Feng Dan Chen*

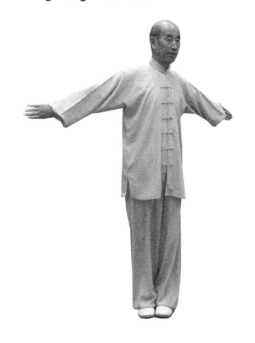

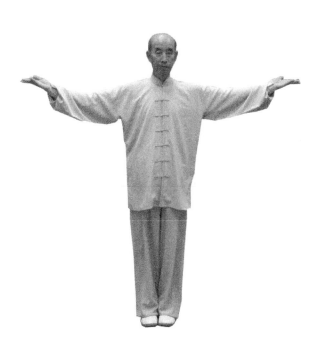

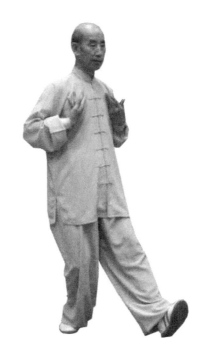

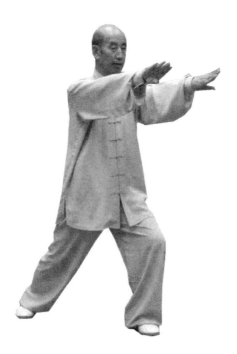

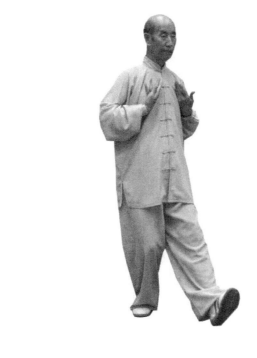

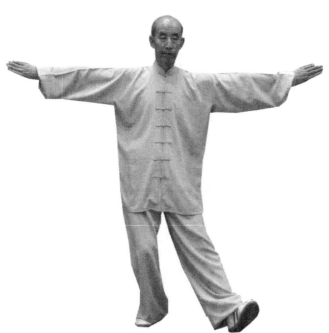

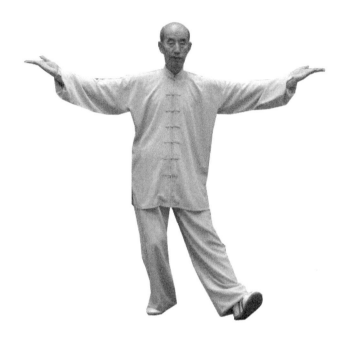

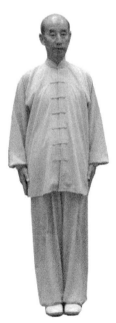

Eighth movement: The ancient sage strokes his beard

老翁拂髯 *Lao Weng Fu Ran*

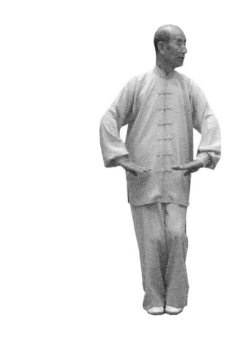

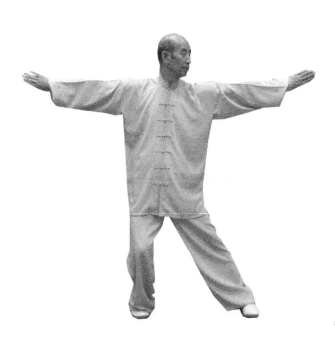

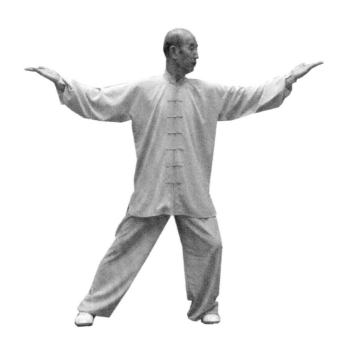

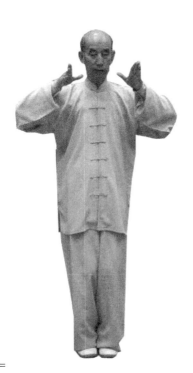
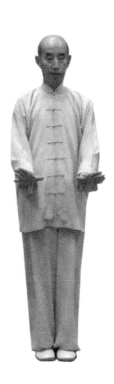

Closing

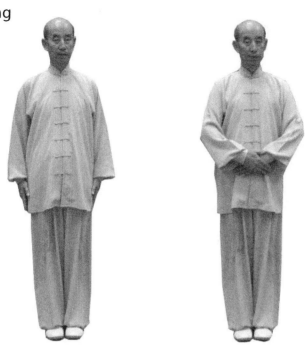

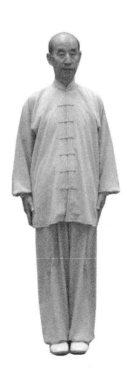

PART 2

Commentary by Dr André Perret

INTRODUCTION: *DAO YIN BAO JIAN GONG*

導 *Dao*: the way, the path, the principle, i.e. the implementation of the unity of *Yin* and *Yang*

引 *Yin*: to shoot, but also to guide, as on the archery range where it is necessary to unite the attention, the breathing and the precision of the movement

Dao Yin: a Taoist physical practice that combines the attention, breathing and precision of movement to attain a perfection of union of *Yin* and *Yang* within oneself

保 *Bao*: to protect

健 *Jian*: to strengthen

功 *Gong*: exercises

The literal translation of the title of this sequence is therefore '*Dao Yin* exercises to protect and strengthen'. As the sequence aims to protect and strengthen the health, it is commonly referred to as '*Dao Yin* to benefit the health in general', or '*Dao Yin* for general health'. Thus the action of this sequence is comprehensive when compared to other *Dao Yin Yang Sheng Gong* sequences that have a more specific action on one of the bodily systems (kidney, spleen, heart, etc.).

The comprehensiveness of its action on the health and in the prevention and treatment of illness explains why this sequence is known and used by most practitioners of the *Dao Yin Yang Sheng Gong* system.

That said, the importance of the two terms – *Bao*, to protect, and *Jian*, to strengthen – chosen by Professor Zhang Guangde, needs to be emphasised because they are the theoretical basis and the technical guide of each movement.

This sequence has a very soft, fluid and light appearance. It seems to be easy to perform, but beneath this softness the work is very deep, with powerful internal strength. As is often the case, something that seems easy, is, in fact, not as simple as it looks. A high level of technical precision is required in order to comply with the characteristics, as defined by Professor Zhang Guangde below:

- The close association of 形 *Xing* (the form, posture), and 意 *Yi* (the idea, intention), with the emphasis on *Yi*.

- The harmonisation of the movement and the breathing, with the emphasis on the breathing.

- Relaxes the entire body, producing relaxed and attractive postures and movements.

- When a movement involves rotation, the postures that form the movement will also contain twisting or winding.

- Contracts and relaxes the *Gu Dao* (the anus); coordinate this action with the breathing.

- The movements are gentle, slow, balanced, harmonious, and follow one to another in a continuous manner.

RULES AND PRINCIPLES IN THE MOVEMENTS

If certain rules for the conduct and coordination of movements are respected, then this practice will provide a very different experience from ordinary physical exercise.

First, it is necessary to differentiate between *Dong* (movement) and *Zuo* (posture). Movement and posture are different. For the movements; the rules and principles must be learned and followed. The postures require the correct forms and shapes. If these requirements are not achieved, the method is distorted and becomes ineffective.

This concept – respecting the rules and finding the form – is the basis of good practice. Even 20 years of experience is insufficient to attain quality if the principles have not been followed and if the posture is not correct. The main concern for the good teacher is to ensure that the practitioner respects the rules and the shape in the movements and postures. When we know and follow the rules and principles, then even with only ten minutes practice we can understand and feel something. This notion is an essential requirement of the sequence.

The aim of this commentary is to help practitioners to comply with these rules and principles through the introduction of technical details, in the main taken from seminars taught by Professor Zhang Guangde. Taken in conjunction with the details of this sequence, they assist the practitioner to make more rapid progress and to experience the subtle and deep sensations associated with this practice.

PREPARATION[9]

In order to stand upright and straight, with the feet together, it is essential to push the top of the head (i.e. the point *Bai Hui* (GV20), located at the midpoint of a line joining the tops of both ears) upward. At the same time, the shoulders are dropped. The shoulders should not be 'closed',[10] pushed upward or forward.

---

9   This preparation posture, 'Standing, find the axis (*Zhong Jian*)', is described in detail in the book *Dao Yin Yang Sheng Gong Foundation Sequences 2*, Singing Dragon.

10   The point *Yun Men* (Lu2) (cloud gate) is found beneath the clavicle, near the shoulder. When the shoulders are raised and pushed forward, this point is hidden in a depression. However, raising *Bai Hui* and lowering the shoulders stretches this area, and the point *Yun Men* reappears. Then it can be said that the 'cloud gate' is open. The term 'cloud' represents intense suffering, sadness, as well as illness. Opening the cloud gate is the beginning of healing. In fact, when there is no suffering, the posture changes naturally. Conversely, modifying the posture increases muscle tone and promotes relaxation.

This poor posture is often produced by weakness in the thoracic spine, producing a rounded back. Pushing *Bai Hui* upward stretches the spine and lowers the shoulders. Alternatively, lowering the shoulders (without rounding the back) produces a feeling of pushing *Bai Hui* upwards. In this way, the movements of ascent (*Bai Hui*) and descent (shoulders) are linked.

Cross the hands and place them on the surface of *Dan Tian*.[11] The left hand (*Yang*) is underneath for both men and women in order to stimulate the movement (*Yang*) of blood and energy.

The poem: 'It is night, everything is silent...'

Even during the daytime, this phrase encourages us to seek complete calmness. In order to calm the mind the attention is focused on the area of *Dan Tian*. Then we are not looking at anything, not listening to anything; we are not aware of odours: this is what is meant by '*close the seven openings of the face.*'

The tongue touches the palate to form the *magpie bridge.*[12] The breathing is fine, deep and slow.

When these three principles (the position of the body, the state of mind and the quality of the breathing) are well established and united, the body seems to become very light (like the bird referred to in the poem, flying to the distant clouds). These three principles must always be present in the practice of *Dao Yin*.

---

11 Described in detail in *Dao Yin Yang Sheng Gong Foundation Sequences 1 and 2*, Singing Dragon.

12 Also described in detail in *Dao Yin Yang Sheng Gong Foundation Sequences 1 and 2*, Singing Dragon.

FIRST MOVEMENT: REGULATE THE BREATH

Key points

- Maintain stability when shifting the bodyweight. For example, when stepping with the left foot, place the weight on the right foot, bending the knees. Create stability through this strong 'rooting' connection with the ground, and then move the left foot. Only when the left foot is completely on the ground should the pelvis be moved horizontally between the two feet, then vertically as the legs straighten, thus equalising the bodyweight.

- To lift the arms, first push *Bai Hui* (GV20): drawing up the *Qi* with *Bai Hui* raises the back of the wrist. However, to raise *Bai Hui* correctly, it is essential to lower the shoulders and raise the tongue to the palate to form *Que Qiao* (the magpie bridge).

- Bending the knees lowers the buttocks and causes the arms to descend. The arms do not move independently. If the legs and arms move separately, there is no energetic link. To create this energetic connection between the upper and lower parts of the body, slightly lower the shoulders before bending the knees: a physical, energetic and expiratory sensation appears on the sides of the chest, linking the upper and lower part of the body during the movement of descent.[13] Then, the lowering of the body by bending the knees is felt and is transmitted to the hands. The movement of the knees, hips and shoulders enables the descent of the arms.

- In order to push the hands, first the knees need to bend, then, raising the trunk and pushing *Bai Hui* produces the movement that lifts the wrists and the arms. These sensations

---

13 For this sensation to appear, the body must be held upright by raising *Bai Hui*.

must be experienced in order to be confident that you are practising the techniques properly.

- When lowering the hands to waist height, the elbows descend but must not touch the side of the body or the chest. Maintain a space between the elbow and belly.

- The distance between the hands should be more or less shoulder width; it can be a little less, but to bring them too close will impede the movement of energy.

- When bending the knees a little more to push the hands forward, earth energy can be experienced entering *Lao Gong* (HP8). When the hands are lifted by the backs of the wrists, *Lao Gong* acts like a mouth, sucking in this energy.[14]

- The knees advance a little when bending, and the bodyweight moves slightly forward and thus pushes the heels of the hands. The palms face forward when pushing, but face downward when the wrists move upward.

- At the moment of the change from lowering to rising, and from exhalation to inhalation, there is a subtle coordination between the movement of the wrist and the movement of the bodyweight from the heel to the ball of the foot.

- The movement leaves the shoulder, spreads to the elbow and then the wrist. It is like a wave composed of three movements flowing one from the other in succession and without pause. The beauty of the movement is found in the creation of this wave, always in harmony with the circular movement of *Tai Ji*. Even though the area of concentration is *Dan Tian*, there must still be an awareness of the movement in the arms travelling like a wave: the shoulder, elbow, wrist.

---

14 In the practice of *Dao Yin*, earth energy (*Yin*) is utilised to obtain vitality. Of course, the collection of *Yang* energy is also used in *Dao Yin*, but the collection of *Yin* energy is equally important. In Chinese Buddhist temples, the Buddha is shown with bare feet to collect the *Yin* energy of the earth. This is why the great saints are often referred to as 'bare footed'.

- Just as in descending, when rising the shoulders should remain lowered in order to maintain the energetic link between the upper and lower parts of the body.

- There is also a principle that should be respected at the end of the movement, when closing the feet and lowering the arms: to lower the arms, push *Bai Hui* upward. In practice this means the movement of straightening the body must be well coordinated with the downward movement of the arms. Pushing *Bai Hui* upward causes the shoulders to lower and therefore the arms descend. The main movement is pushing *Bai Hui*, which straightens the body; the secondary movement is the lowering of the arms. This principle applies to all the movements when bringing the feet together.

Therapeutic action

As the title of this movement indicates, its objective is to regulate the breathing. According to the theory of *Yang Sheng*, i.e. how to maintain and improve your life, above all things, it is breathing that nourishes life. But inhalation and exhalation are like the mountains and the sea, and a balance between them is necessary for their effectiveness. This movement appears to be simple, but is actually challenging and subtle, because it relies entirely on deep, soft, regular and balanced breathing. The movement is obviously observed externally, but the purpose of this external movement is to assist the internal work produced by our energy and breath.

We must therefore respect the principles for the raising and lowering of the body and the arms. Furthermore, the harmonisation of the breathing and circular movements at the level of the feet, knees, *Dan Tian*, chest, elbows, shoulders and wrists is necessary. All these movements, which originate in *Dan Tian*, amplify the circular movement of the hands. Externally, we see the hands move, but the real work is internal, and must be emphasised in correct proper practice.

The area of concentration is *Dan Tian*. In fact, this area needs to become dynamic in order to generate the rest of the sequence. The quality of the succeeding movements depends on the energetic state of *Dan Tian*. If vitality is lacking in *Dan Tian*, the rest of the movements will be lifeless. *Dan Tian* is like the source of a river – if the source is weak, then the rest of the river is weak; if the source is abundant, then the river flows easily. Thus, the main therapeutic action of this movement is to strengthen central energy and consolidate original energy.

A further therapeutic action is produced by the movement of the wrists that enables the collection of *Yin* (earth energy) and frees the *Yin* and *Yang* meridians.[15]

---

15 Regulating the breathing enables the linking of these two therapeutic actions. The circular breathing movements of *Dan Tian* are transmitted in turn to the chest, shoulders, elbows and hands. Each movement is separate, but together they provide capacity in the breathing and breadth in the gestures.

SECOND MOVEMENT: PUSH THE BOAT DOWNSTREAM

Key points

- To 'place the hands on the boat', turn the trunk 45° to the left; raise the arms by the backs of the wrists, turn the trunk slightly to the right, then again to the left, and step to the left diagonal, onto the left heel. When stepping out with the left foot, draw the hands back in front of the chest at shoulder height. This is an example of linking the 'outward' movement (the foot) and 'inward' (the hands). The movement of the trunk generates the movement of the hands: this kind of technique is known as *Shen Fa*.[16] Turning the trunk to the left raises the hands; turning it to the right draws the hands back; returning the trunk to the left moves the hands in front of the chest. When the hands are at shoulder height, drop the elbows.

- When forming 左虚步 *Zuo Xu Bu* (the 'empty' step), it is important to turn the pelvis 45°, bend the hips and lower the buttocks; the upper body remains upright and the lumbar muscles relaxed.

- The most visible element of this particular exercise is the movement of the hands as they push the boat: as they advance, the arms and hands move a little closer to each other. When the hands are forward, the shoulders and elbows are lowered, and the wrists are bent.

- However, the 'boat' is not 'pushed' by the movement of the arms, but by the movement of the lumbar region. When the front heel is placed on the ground, the weight remains on the back foot. The root of pushing the boat lies in the back heel and the loins. This root initiates the movement of the arms.

---

16 身 *Shen*: the body, 法 *Fa*: method.

In order to lower the hands it is necessary to lower the pelvis, bending the hips and lowering the buttocks: the power comes from the heel and is transmitted to the loins. The power from the heel and loins causes the movement of the pelvis and the trunk, then the elbows, wrists and hands. Finally, the internal strength is manifested in the hands. To maintain the connected movement of the heel and the loins, keep the shoulders low.

- When practising this movement, develop an awareness of when the rotation of the trunk generates the rising and the placement of hands before pushing, then feel the power in the heel and loins as it pushes the boat. Lower the hands when bending the hips to root the heel, then push with the heel and the loins to advance the hands, fingers upward. These techniques give great strength to the movement.

- Furthermore, when beginning to push the boat, simultaneously lower the bodyweight. When pushing the boat the pelvis must not be lifted. In order to use less strength at this point, there is a natural tendency to raise the pelvis, but this is not correct. Although lowering the bodyweight is more difficult, it is much better. In this way, we can experience both lightness within the movement and the strength of internal power. Bending the hips, lowering the buttocks and the bodyweight is the most subtle and difficult part of this exercise. It requires a great deal of practice to achieve this and experience this quality within the movement.

- When the boat has been pushed, the palms are forward, and the back leg straight,[17] but it is essential that the buttocks are lowered and the body is upright.

---

17   The back leg may be slightly bent, because if the knee is too straight, energy does not flow well. It can be said that even in tension there must be a little flexibility.

- Then relax the wrists, the palms face downward, and draw the pelvis back to move the hands. It is always the movement of the pelvis that generates the movement of the hands.

- In element 1, with the feet still together, turn the body at the right moment to bring back the hands: turn slightly right, then left again. In elements 3 and 5, the rotation begins after having brought the bodyweight onto the back foot. All these small details increase the subtlety of the practice.

- In element 8, bring the pelvis back, retaining the 45° rotation to the left, then turn the pelvis to bring the hands forward, bring the foot back, then straighten the knees, pushing *Bai Hui* and lowering the arms. It is important to coordinate the movement of straightening the body and lowering the arms. The movement of the arms results from the movement of the body.

Therapeutic action

The place of concentration is *Lao Gong* (HP8). This point, in the palm of the hand, is an ancient *Shu* (spring) point. It is very sensitive to opening, and is a major point for the gathering of external energy. The circular movements of the arms and hands stimulate the *Yuan* (source) points and also the *Lao Gong* points. This action strengthens the heart and lungs, regulates the Triple Heater, humidifies the large intestine preventing constipation, and also acts on masses, tumours and haemorrhoids.

The act of pushing stretches *Lao Gong* and it releases energy. When the hands are drawn back, *Lao Gong* is in a hollow formed by the palm; then it draws in external energy. These actions follow the rhythm of the breathing.

THIRD MOVEMENT: CARRY THE SUN AND MOON ON THE SHOULDERS

This beautiful movement is often used in Chinese traditional performances. It is very simple, but the body must not be too tense.

Here it is necessary to re-emphasise the importance of the rules in the practice because they once again provide the key to the movement. Knowing and understanding the rules leads to knowing and understanding the method, because the construction of the method is based on these principles. Frequently, practitioners develop attractive movements but fail to apply the rules. Ultimately this leads to empty practice, with no internal component. It is not necessary to be Chinese to achieve a high level of practice; everyone can get there, but only by applying the rules and principles.

Key points

- Element 1: the movement begins with a 90° rotation of the trunk combined with a rotation of the hands, bringing the backs of the hands against the thighs. Then, when the rotation of the trunk is complete, the arms are lifted, palms upward. When the arms are raised, they must be aligned so that, when viewed in profile, the rear hand cannot be seen. Without pausing, push *Bai Hui* and open the chest to generate a movement of external rotation from the shoulders to the hands. The movement of the arms must be symmetrical and balanced. The hands remain a little higher than the shoulders, while the shoulders are relaxed and the elbows are dropped to below shoulder level.

- Element 2: on returning, when the trunk has rotated 45°, this is the point at which to begin the rotation of the wrists, not before or after. The rotation of the wrist is very important to stimulate all the *Yuan* (source) points. It is accompanied by a small and light circular movement of the wrist and elbow.

It is said in the *Nei Jing* that lung and heart diseases manifest themselves as abnormal sensations in the elbow where the *He* points of the heart and lung are found. This movement of the elbow can help to treat lung and heart diseases.

- The gaze is connected to the movement: look at the rear hand throughout the movement, then, when lowering the hands, look forward.

- This movement is not easy. It must be done with fluidity and with the rhythm of the music, without pausing. If there is a pause when the hands are raised, palms upward, then it becomes difficult to match the rhythm thereafter.

Therapeutic action

The concentration is on *Ming Men* (GV4) (gate of vitality), the source of reproduction and growth. This point is located between the kidneys and stores the subtle essence related to sexuality and reproduction. It is the source of original *Yin* and *Yang* energy. The rotation of the body frees the bladder meridians and the governing vessel (GV) (five pathways found in the back).

The point *Ming Men* is particularly stimulated during rotations of the trunk. In this movement, the lumbar rotation generates the movement of the hands.

FOURTH MOVEMENT: THE GREAT BIRD SPREADS ITS WINGS

Key points

- It is important to be aware of and to express the essential form within the posture. In this movement the essential form is the circle formed by the arms. This circle represents the *Tai Ji*.

- At the end of the third movement (Carry the sun and moon on the shoulders), bring the hands in front of *Dan Tian*, palms upward; this represents holding the *Tai Ji* and thus the arms form a circle. *Tai Ji* gave birth to *Yin* and *Yang*: when making the step (*Kai Bu*), *Yin* and *Yang* appear in the movement. The stationary right foot is *Yin*, the left foot that moves is *Yang*. When the feet are brought together again, we return to the *Tai Ji*.

- In order to carry the *Tai Ji* correctly, the circle shape must be maintained, the shoulders and elbows dropped, so that the palms are naturally turned upward. Keep a space of about 10cm between the fingers, and 10cm between the hands and the pelvis. The chest is slightly hollowed to conserve energy.

- When the hands are above the head, the arms form the *Tai Ji* circle; the tips of the middle fingers should be vertically in line with the *Jian Yu* points (LI15) on the shoulder.

- When drawing the bodyweight back, fold the hips to move the weight on to the back foot and fill the loins. Lift the toes of the front foot to stretch *Tai Xi* (Kid3), the *Yuan* point of the kidney.

- When raising the arms, it is always the backs of the wrists that lead the movement. The shoulders remain lowered, but the chest opens forward. This movement is very graceful, imitating the wings of the great bird *Peng*. However, to 'fly' further and higher, the details of the technique must be mastered: pushing *Bai Hui* causes the extension of the knees and therefore the lifting of the trunk, and it is the lifting of the trunk that produces the raising of the wrists. The starting point is not the knee; it is the pushing of *Bai Hui*.

- At the end of the movement, in order to return the hands and straighten the legs, pushing *Bai Hui* initiates and controls the movement. The movements of the knees and arms are the result of the action of pushing *Bai Hui*.

Therapeutic action

The area of concentration is *Dan Tian*. The importance of the *Tai Ji* circle within the posture and the requirement to push *Bai Hui* have been emphasised, but it must also be remembered that *Dan Tian* is the source of movement both from the interior to the exterior and vice versa. Placing the concentration at the level of *Dan Tian* enables us to feel the internal origin of the movement. This sensation is enhanced by the breathing (abdominal or reverse abdominal) and by the alternate stretching and compression in this area. This combination of mental, respiratory and physical action amplifies the movement of *Qi* and provides a deep stimulation of the zone of *Dan Tian*.

A further therapeutic effect of this movement is to regulate the Triple Heater. The Triple Heater meridian, *Shou Shao Yang*, begins on the tip of the ring finger, travels up the *Yang* (outside) face of the arm and across the shoulder. A branch returns into the trunk and connects the 'three burners': upper, middle and lower. The main route continues to the head. When the hands are raised, the 'well' point, *Guan Chong* (TH1), is the highest. This posture clears the route of the meridian; blood and energy then flow freely from the top downward, as water flows down a mountain. Finally, the movement of the wrist provides a specific stimulation of the *Yuan* point *Yang Chi* (TH4).

Then all the organs and entrails are released, because the Triple Heater connects the 'three burners': the upper burner houses the lung and the heart, the middle burner the stomach and spleen and the lower burner the kidney and liver. The stretching of the chest and abdomen facilitates this action.

FIFTH MOVEMENT: LIFT THE GREAT STONE WITH POWER

Within Chinese culture, stones are regarded as significant in a variety of ways. Usually, the stones referred to are large and extremely heavy. In addition to its size and weight, the stone in the title also has a spirit, similar to the sacred animals in Chinese culture.

There is a Chinese legend that refers to this particular stone. Chi You, the leader of a minority group in ancient times, travelled to Tai Shan, a mountain sacred to the Taoists. To prove his great strength, he threw several heavy stones. However, a woman named Nu Wa threw a large red stone even further than Chi You. This was the stone of Tai Shan that possessed a spirit. Thus, the power of the spirit surpassed that of purely physical force.

In traditional Chinese houses, a very heavy stone supporting the building is often found on each side of the main door. Of course, these stones are naturally very strong, solid objects, but according to tradition, their strength also comes from their spirits. The stones may be arranged in different ways according to the personality of the family and the character of the house. Over time, this representation of the physical and spiritual strength of the stones has been replaced by two stone lions placed at the entrance to the house for its protection.

Key points

- In this movement, as implied in the title, the great stone is not moved by physical strength alone, but rather through strength of mind, the idea and intent. In technique, this movement is quite similar to the movement 'Sit three times to connect with the earth' found in *Yi Jin Jing*. But *Yi Jin Jing*, a traditional sequence for strengthening the muscles, is somewhat in the martial arts style – i.e. it uses physical force. *Dao Yin*, on the other hand, uses energy and the mind.

This is one of the fundamental differences between *Dao Yin* and martial arts. As it is produced by the mind and not by physical force, the movement is absolutely relaxed and the arms are more extended, the external movement is broader and lighter, as the real work is internal. Thus we can see that these two methods are very different. *Yi Jin Jing* is one of the foundations in the technique of martial arts, and to a large extent it utilises muscular strength. Here, in *Dao Yin*, we work with the energy and the mind: it is by pushing *Bai Hui* (that the stone is able to be lifted). In spite of the differences, both systems apply the same rules and principles of movement.

- In order to descend, maintaining the body upright and pushing *Bai Hui*, first slightly drop the shoulders to create an energetic link between the upper and lower parts of the body. Then, descend simply by bending the knees, which draws the trunk and arms downward, the arms not changing position relative to the body. It is this internal energy that leads the movement, not the arms. The hands will move towards the body only when the pelvis has reached its lowest point. In this way, the movement arises in the tranquility of the concentration. The movement does not come from the exterior. In reality, if we are willing to open ourselves to the sensations of energy and be guided by them, then it becomes easy. Slightly dropping the shoulders at the beginning of the movement creates this feeling of the descending of the energy within the body. When the body lowers, energy naturally also descends. In the practice of *Dao Yin* the aim is to feel this energy descending, allow it to happen and let it become that which creates the movement.

- At the beginning of the movement, when stepping sideways, the coordination is a little different from the usual. As the foot moves, the hands rise up to chest level, then pushing *Bai Hui* and raising the body draws the hands upward and outward.

- In *Ma Bu* (horseriding posture), the feet are parallel, spaced about three foot lengths apart, and the pelvis descends as low as individually possible without pushing out the buttocks – the aim is that the thighs should be parallel to the ground, with the hips bent at 90°. The knees do not go beyond the tips of the toes, and it is especially important that the body is upright. This posture must be very strong in order to 'lift the stone' effortlessly with the arms. Of course, in case of difficulty, the step can be a little narrower and the body a little higher, but the feet must be parallel, toes pointed forward and the body upright.

- Keeping the body upright and pushing *Bai Hui* upward provides free space within the body for the circulation of energy. If blood and energy flow freely without blockages, there will be no illness. It is said that when energy circulates harmoniously, the body is at peace; when its movement is disturbed, illness results; when it stops, life ends. So maintaining an upright body nourishes energy.

  In this movement there are further rules to be observed:

  ○ The movements of the arms and legs must be connected: the hands rise because the body rises; the hands lower because the body lowers.

  ○ Rising is the result of pushing *Bai Hui* upwards.

  ○ To begin to open the hands, open the chest.

  ○ Complete the opening of the hands by describing an arc of a circle with them.

  ○ Before descending, drop the shoulders to unify the movement of the pelvis and the arms. The strength of the lowering of the pelvis is then transmitted to the hands.

  ○ Lowering is the result of bending the knees.

- When the body is descending, release the elbows.

- Before lifting the stone, both hands move in front of and below the level of the knees.

- At the end of the movement, push *Bai Hui* to lower the arms.

Therapeutic action

The concentration is on *Dan Tian*. In this movement, the strength (physical, energetic, respiratory, and mental) finds its source in *Dan Tian*.[18] This force increases throughout the movement to strengthen the energetic transformation at the level of *Dan Tian*.

---

18 See *Dao Yin Yang Sheng Gong Foundation Sequences 1 and 2*, Singing Dragon.

SIXTH MOVEMENT: PUSH THE WINDOW TO LOOK AT THE MOON

Key points

This is the most difficult movement of the sequence, and its complex structure contains different elements that require detailed explanation.

- Slightly rotate the body to the left, the arms rising, the backs of the hands facing each other. When the arms have reached 45°, begin an external rotation of the left arm to turn the palm forward. Continue to lift the hands, left arm extended, the right hand remaining near to the body, wrist relaxed. Look at the movement of the left hand. When the left arm reaches 90°, i.e. at shoulder height, it is fully extended, palm forward. The right forearm and elbow are also at shoulder height, with the right elbow bent. The right hand, palm forward, is at chest level, in front of the left shoulder and slightly higher than the left elbow. In this way, the energy is not blocked in the chest. Frequently, there is a tendency to bring the right hand to far to the left side, which then obstructs the energy in the chest. To avoid this, at the end of the raising of the arms, the right elbow should be pulled slightly to the right to bring the right hand in front of the chest. This posture will enable the opening of the chest, which in the remainder of the movement will result in the drawing of the hands to the right. Look at the left hand.

- Beginning with the feet together, turn the trunk to the right, moving the body weight on to the right foot and drawing the hands towards the face. The moving hands describe a semicircle but remain below head height as they pass in front of the face. The gaze follows the left hand. When both hands pass in front of the face, fingers upward, the gaze changes to follow the right hand. The body continues to turn, and then lowers by bending the hip and the right knee and stepping out with the left foot. The lowering of the body causes the hands to also lower. In this posture the trunk is well turned to the right, the right arm is extended but rounded, the right wrist is cocked and shoulder height. The fingers of both hands point upward, the fingers of the left hand level with the right elbow. The left (rear) leg is extended, the right knee and hip flexed. The shoulders must be dropped and the buttocks lowered.

- Pivot on the left foot, moving the heel to guide the point of the foot forward. The left knee then flexes slightly and the pelvis turns forward. Then relax the wrists and turn the left palm forward. The rotation of the trunk causes the left shoulder and elbow to lower: the left hand is placed before the chest near to the right shoulder. These three elements need to be carried out with harmony, continuity and circularity: the movement of the foot and the pelvis creates the movement of the trunk and the hands. Both palms are forward, fingers pointing to the right. To draw the pelvis back, the weight moves on to the bent left leg, and the right leg extends. When moving the bodyweight the hands remain parallel to the ground, palms forward. Then, when the bodyweight is solidly on the left foot, step diagonally back with the right foot. The hands remain in place. Always look at the right hand.

- Bend the knees, and then 'push the window'. According to individual ability, it is acceptable here to form the higher posture *Xie Bu* (where the buttocks rest on the back heel) rather than *Pa Gen Bu* (twisted roots posture), but whichever posture is chosen, the thighs must be pressed one against the other. The movement of the hands is generated by the rotation of the trunk; for this to happen, the shoulders must not be raised. The gaze initially follows the right hand and then passes on to the left hand. When 'pushing the window to look at the moon', do not incline the trunk or the head. Both hands are almost vertically in line with each other, fingers forward, the right elbow is close to the body and pushes in order to turn the trunk and advance the right hand.

- Rotate the wrists before lowering the hands. Dropping the elbows, the wrists draw an arc to guide the palms downward. Dropping the elbows enables the energy to descend to *Dan Tian*. Without the lowering of the elbows and the rotating of the wrists, the energy does not descend. Dropping the shoulders initiates the lowering of the elbows, which in turn generates the wrist rotation. Turn the trunk to move the hands. The fingers are then pointing forward. Lower the hands, forward and down, palms downward. Then straighten the body and raise the arms to the right with the same arm's internal rotation as in element 1. Close the feet when the arms are at 45° and the arms are beginning the external rotation. Continue to raise the hands as in element 1. Then continue the rest of the movement in the other direction.

- This sixth movement of the sequence is performed to the left and right twice, in two sets of eight elements. However, in the second set of eight, it is necessary to add the closing movement of bringing the arms in front of the body, standing up and finally lowering the arms. Therefore in order to maintain the breathing pattern, element 7 must be performed more quickly than before, and include the action of 'pushing the window to look at the moon' – i.e. element 7 is a combination of the previous elements 7 and 8, and is performed while inhaling. The final element 8 (exhaling) then begins with lowering the elbows and hands in front of the body. Begin to stand up, raising the hands. Bring the feet together when both hands are at shoulder height, then straighten the legs, pushing *Bai Hui* upward and lowering the hands. In this way, you are ready to begin the seventh movement of the sequence without being out of breath.

- The absence of shortness of breath is one of the major differences between Western sport and *Dao Yin*. Here the body is hot, but we are never breathless because the movement follows and assists the breathing. In the practice of *Dao Yin*, physical strength is at the service of the energy. Most Western sports require considerable physical effort and therefore a lot of energy is expended, but this is not a mutually supportive combination of strength and energy. This is why we sweat and become exhausted. In *Dao Yin*, the practitioner descends, rises, advances, retreats: we derive benefit from the movements of the body. We make the gestures in order to experience our bodies.

Therapeutic action

What is the significance of the phrase, 'push the window to look at the moon'? It indicates that in the practice of *Dao Yin* we may experience a union and harmony between ourselves and nature. This same concept applies to the poem of preparation: 'It is night, everything is silent...' At night, the moon is regarded as *Tai Yin*. *Tai* means 'very', so the moon is thought of as extremely *Yin*. It is referred to as *Tai Yin* because it derives its brightness from the sun, *Tai Yang*, reflecting sunlight, being unable to produce its own light. *Yin* represents absolute calm, and it is this state of calm that we seek through our practice. A Chinese poem says, 'Find calmness like the moon on an Autumn night'. This is true tranquillity and stillness. But within the movement, there is also calmness, and this calm is like a weeping willow caressed by the breeze. Consequently, although this particular movement is physically difficult, we must endeavour to perform it in a state of great tranquillity, using the great symbol of calmness, the moon, to help us.

The highest level of *Dao Yin* practice aims to achieve virtue, clarity and order. Three sentences summarise the basis of Taoism and traditional Chinese thought, i.e. the essential concept of the union of man with nature by means of these three qualities:

Man is united with Heaven and Earth through virtue.
He unites with the sun and the moon through clarity.
He connects with the natural order of things.

Heaven and earth give life to the 10,000 beings. This is the greatest of the virtues. Mankind's own virtue must be great, like that of heaven and earth. Standing between heaven and earth, man connects with them through heavenly and earthly virtues. This connection must always be present in the practice of *Dao Yin*.

In practising *Dao Yin*, we connect with the clarity and light of the sun and the moon. We must reflect this clarity in ourselves and in our practice.

The natural rhythms, in particular, the rhythms of the four seasons, form the basis of order in life. Human beings adapt and change according to the changing seasons. The internal rhythms of *Dao Yin* connect with these external natural rhythms.

The sixth movement is complex because it combines several actions:

- strong stimulation of all the *Yuan* points at the ankles and wrists

- stretching and rotating the limbs, thus stimulating all the meridians

- rotating the trunk and stimulating *Ming Men* (GV4)

- opening and closing the chest and stimulating the three burners

- stretching and contracting the abdomen and stimulating *Dan Tian*.

This exercise is very comprehensive and produces considerable movement of energy. This is why it must be performed in a state of complete calmness, established through technical precision and mental relaxation, enabling us to perform the difficult movements with fluency.

The concentration is on *Lao Gong* (HP8), which is also the place of exchange and harmonisation between the movement of internal energy and the energy of the universe, represented here by the moon.

SEVENTH MOVEMENT: BRUSH THE DUST INTO THE WIND

Key points

- The movements of the feet and the pelvis are the same as in the second movement, 'Push the boat downstream'.

- To turn the trunk to the left, first turn slightly to the right.

- To rise, first descend.

Additional details

- Element 1: in this movement, the most difficult gesture is the rotation of the arms. The key is to know exactly how and when to do it correctly, i.e. it must be linked to the movements of the trunk. The internal rotation of the arms links with the turning left of the body, the external rotation links with the right turn, and turning again to the left draws in the arms in external rotation. In order to raise and open the arms, it is essential to push *Bai Hui* upward and open the chest. When the arms are spread with the palms upward, they should be naturally extended, i.e. the elbows are slightly lowered. Bending the knees allows the pelvis to descend, the left foot to step out, and also draws the elbows down. The hands pass in front of the face, descend, and then press lightly on the chest with the inside edge. It is the movement of the elbows that produces the movement of the hands. The movement of the feet and hands must be coordinated: the heel should touch the ground at the same moment as the hands arrive at the chest.

- Element 2: in order to move the body weight into *Zuo Gong Bu* (the 'bow' step), use the same rules of movement found in the second movement, 'Push the boat downstream'.

Lower the bodyweight before pushing it forward. It would be easier to move forward without lowering the bodyweight, but the result would be a posture that is too light and unstable. Lowering the centre of gravity enables the body to be grounded and to move forward firmly. Rotating the trunk consolidates this rooting. Look for the basis of this rooting in the heel (bending at the hips to lower the buttocks), and use the lower back as the pivot. In this way the energy and power spreads progressively until it reaches the fingers. This progression begins in the heel and moves through the loins to the chest and from there to the hands. When the bodyweight moves forward (throwing away the dust), the hands turn the palms outward, slightly higher than shoulder height.

- Element 3: to move the body back into *Zuo Xu Bu* ('empty' step), again use the same rules as in the second movement, 'Push the boat downstream'.

- Element 7: draw back, then turn the trunk forward, bringing the hands to the chest; draw the hands down the body, then raise the arms to either side, still in internal rotation, then externally rotate them to bring the palms upward. The arms are naturally extended, at shoulder height.

- Element 8: bring the hands towards the face and bring the feet together. Lower the hands, palms facing the floor, at the same time pushing *Bai Hui* to straighten the legs.

- This description of elements 7 and 8 differs slightly from the translation of the original text (above). On the instruction of Professor Zhang Guangde, element 7 (and thus also the inhalation) should be considered to end when both arms are extended, palms upward, and not when the hands are touching the chest.

- At the end of this seventh movement, the arms descend in front of the body, but there should be no pause in the movement of the hands as they begin the eighth movement.

Therapeutic action

In this movement, we 'brush' the dust in accordance with the wind, not against the wind: we use the strength of the light wind to assist us to clear the dust. For the Chinese, brushing dust from clothing is done with the back of the hand. The movement of the hands takes advantage of the force of the airflow: as the hands move backward, the dust is blown from our hands, using the airflow coming from the front. The objective of this movement is to purify the mind: it is both a physical and psychological exercise.

Before drawing the forearms down the trunk, make an external rotation (supination) of the arms. This maximum rotation releases the three *Yin* and three *Yang* meridians – lungs, heart, heart protector, large intestine, small intestine and Triple Heater.

The flexing of the wrists, which occurs when the elbows open and draw back, stimulates the *Yuan* points of the wrists.

It is important to turn and lower the bodyweight to produce a stronger stimulation on the heel and ankle. The six *Yuan* points of the foot, distributed around the ankle area, connect to the organs and viscera – liver, spleen, kidney, stomach, gallbladder and bladder.

The pressure produced at the toes as they press against the floor stimulates the 'well' points. These are points that can produce a burst of energy and blood. We stimulate this energetic area to stimulate the propulsion and circulation of the blood and energy. Thus, by the self-massage on the heel, ankle and toe involved in this exercise, we improve the functioning of the organs related to the meridians concerned.

EIGHTH MOVEMENT: THE ANCIENT SAGE SMOOTHS HIS BEARD

Additional details

- Element 1: bodyweight must first be stabilised on the right foot before stepping sideways with the left foot. When opening the feet, they must remain parallel with the toes pointing forward. When opening the arms sideways with an internal then external rotation, the rotations must be done to the maximum extent possible. The arms must be raised to shoulder level and the elbows slightly lowered at the end of external rotation. When raising the arms in internal rotation, they must be lifted as high as possible (90° is the aim), but without lifting the shoulders. Those whose movement is limited by joint problems should begin the external rotation as soon as the arms have reached their limit, to enable the further raising of the arms to 90°. The rotations of the arms must be coordinated with the movements of the lower body. When the arms rise in internal rotation, open the feet. Then, the external rotation happens as the bodyweight shifts.

- Element 2: bring the hands toward the face while closing the feet. When the feet are together, the hands should have reached ear level, where the 'beard' begins. The fingers point towards each other, but the thumb is opened from the index finger (*Hu Kou*, tiger's mouth). As the hands travel down the 'beard', the thumbs turn forward because of the rotation of the forearms that in turn alter the angle of the wrists. In order to lower the hands, the elbows are gently pushed downward. The hands turn forward because the elbows descend and approach the body, i.e. the orientation of the hands is the result of the movement of the elbows. But when the hands arrive at chest level, there is also a small outward movement of the wrist which pulls the index finger outward, opening the space between it and the thumb, the thumb turning forward and the other fingers also turning outward a little. As the beard is very long and it is difficult to smooth it all against the body, at the end of the movement, we imagine we push it slightly forward. Here, too, the movement of the hands is led by the movement of the elbows, but a light circular motion of the wrists enables the smooth transition between the push and return of the hands. As the hands lower, the legs progressively straighten, generated by pushing *Bai Hui* and lowering the shoulders.

Therapeutic action

This movement is easier because it is the final one. We expend less energy at this point in order to bring the sequence to an end in a state of calmness in harmony with the peaceful flow of *Qi.*

The rotations of the arms, coupled with the movements of the feet and the body, and the stimulation of the wrists, releases all the meridians to facilitate the circulation of *Qi.* It is most important to guide energy to *Dan Tian* when lowering the hands in front of the body while exhaling, when *Qi* is flowing more freely throughout the body. Thus there is total harmony between the interior and the exterior.

This movement requires little effort, and is concerned with regulating the respiration. Because it is physically undemanding, we can give our whole attention to the required reverse abdominal breathing. When inhaling, lower and move the body while drawing in the buttocks and tightening the *Gu Dao* (the anus) to feel *Ming Men* (gate of vitality). When exhaling, the lowering of the shoulders facilitates the lifting of *Bai Hui*, the raising of the body and the lowering of the hands, all of which encourages the descent of the *Qi* to *Dan Tian.*

The movements of the body, breath and energy intersect; they are coordinated and interdependent. Thus, from a very simple, very calm gesture, energy appears. At the end of the exhalation, the light pushing forward of the hands adds a feeling of softness and lightness throughout the body.

This action on the respiration and the *Qi* should be linked with a particular and appropriate mental action: throughout the movement one should imagine being the old sage smoothing his beard. This visualisation encapsulates the wisdom, satisfaction and simplicity found in this exercise.

In the Chinese tradition, the most important thing for an elderly person is to rediscover the heart of a child. This movement creates a visible manifestation of someone whose mind is very clear and simple. As old age is our future, we must give it our attention before it arrives. Traditionally, Chinese thought recognises three periods of childhood in a lifetime. In early childhood, one is truly a child, everything is simple and direct; something is good or not good. The second childhood, when young men and women are more than 18, but nevertheless are not yet quite adult, they still have the simplicity of a child, but are in a period of change. The third childhood corresponds to the elderly person who regains the heart of a child. Maintaining a child's heart is one of the most important elements for good health and wellbeing – old age becomes 'the golden period' of life. Each of the stages of life is important – early childhood and growth, the second childhood, leading to adulthood with its personal, professional and familial fulfilment, but it is the third childhood that is the most important period for health preservation. After experiencing life's trials, the elderly need to know the value of keeping the heart and mind simple and open, and of simplifying daily life.

Unfortunately, the approach of the end of life creates great sadness in many old people. This sadness aggravates already fragile health. However, if the elderly person can, on the other hand, rediscover a childlike joy and simplicity, s/he can enjoy all the benefits of what life has to offer, and will experience a return to a youthful state. Creating this state of mind is one of the key factors in promoting longevity.

So in this exercise we should envisage ourselves as a wise old person with the heart and mind of a child.

There are eight movements in this sequence. The concentration is most often on *Dan Tian*, but also on *Ming Men* (gate of vitality) or *Lao Gong* (palace of labour). This indicates that the main objective is therefore to strengthen original internal energy, although we also gather external, natural energy. In the last movement, we need a very calm, almost meditative mind, in order to preserve this energy.

The International Institute of *Dao Yin Yang Sheng Gong* The School of Professor Zhang Guangde

The International Institute of Dao Yin Yang Sheng Gong (IIDYYSG) is a 'not for profit' association founded in 2004 at the request of Professor Zhang Guangde, the creator of the *Dao Yin Yang Sheng Gong* system. This project was made possible by the active involvement of Dr André Perret and Professor Zhu Mian Sheng, both specialists in Traditional Chinese Medicine, seventh *Duan* of *Dao Yin Yang Sheng Gong*, founders and respectively president and vice president of this association.

OBJECTIVES

- To teach and disseminate *Dao Yin Yang Sheng Gong* in Europe.

- To encourage technical, theoretical and clinical research in this system.

- To train people in the correct knowledge of the techniques and theory of the *Dao Yin Yang Sheng Gong* system.

- To train people to become capable of teaching this method.

- To encourage cultural exchanges concerning health between East and West.

PROGRAMME

In the four years from 2005 to 2009, the IIDYYSG organised training courses in Biarritz for initiation and also the training of teachers in *Dao Yin Yang Sheng Gong*. These courses were directed by Professor Zhang Guangde himself, assisted by his nephew Zhang Jian in the technical demonstrations.

This extensive programme was designed by Professor Zhang Guangde to provide a global understanding and detailed knowledge of his method.

The theoretical and practical teaching programme consisted of 432 hours of training for 29 different sequences of *Dao Yin* and *Yang Sheng Tai Ji*.

More than 500 practitioners from France and other countries benefited from the whole or part of this exceptional teaching programme.

At the end of 2009 as envisaged, Professor Zhang Guangde relinquished his teaching post in Biarritz because of his advancing years, since then the Institute has concerned itself with publications, and with research into *Dao Yin Yang Sheng Gong*.

PUBLICATIONS

Our goal is to offer a quality translation of the associated text for each sequence, written by Zhang Guangde, along with a video presentation by Zhang Guangde and demonstration by Zhang Jian.

All Professor Zhang Guangde's courses and conferences have been filmed and archived.

These archives, as well as numerous debates and discussions on the technical, theoretical and clinical research between the three founders of the IIDYYSG, are the source of the additional comments in this publication.

Zhu Mian Sheng

Born in 1948 in Kunming, Yunnan.

Graduate in Traditional Chinese Medicine of Yunnan and Beijing Universities.

Professor of the Beijing University of Medicine and Chinese Traditional Pharmacopeia.

Associate Professor of the Yunnan University of Traditional Chinese Medicine and the Kunming Institute of Western Medicine.

Senior consultant in Traditional Chinese Medicine.

Graduate in Medical Anthropology from the Faculty of Medicine at the University of Paris 13.

Doctor of Social Sciences at the University of Paris 13.

External expert of AFSSAPS (Agence française de sécurité sanitaire des produits de santé (French Agency for the Safety of Health Products)) for the Chinese Pharmacopoeia.

Practitioner of Traditional Chinese Medicine since 1976.

Teacher of Traditional Chinese Medicine with the Faculty of Medicine, University of Paris 13, since 1989. Director of the Diploma in Traditional Chinese Medicine in this Faculty since 1997.

Member of the office of the World Federation of Medicine and Chinese Traditional Medicine Societies (WFCMS) in Beijing since 2004.

President of the Pan-European Federation of Consultants in Traditional Chinese Medicine (PEFCTCM) since 2002.

Author of numerous books published in China.

Published in France:

- *Breathing and Energy* (medical *Qi Gong*)

- *Know How to Eat to Know How to Live* (Chinese dietetic)

- *Time, Points, Space* (chronoacupuncture).

Author of more than 70 articles in China and elsewhere, in international congresses and international reviews of Traditional Chinese Medicine.

Director of the editorial board of the International Sino-French Prescriptive Nomenclature of Words and Basic Expressions of Chinese Medicine under the direction of the WFCMS.

Co-founder and vice president of the International Institute of Dao Yin Yang Sheng Gong (IIDYYSG) in Biarritz, France, since 2005.

André Perret

Born in 1955 in Bayonne.

Doctorate in Medicine in 1984.

Diploma of Acupuncture of the French School of Acupuncture.

University Degree in Traditional Chinese Medicine.

University Degree in Homeopathy.

University Degree in Osteopathy.

Clinical Exercise Specialist (C.E.S.) of Sports Medicine.

Professor Emeritus of the Yunnan University of Traditional Chinese Medicine.

Practising *Dao Yin Yang Sheng Gong* since 1988 with teachers of Yunnan University Traditional Chinese Medicine, and since 1995 with the teachers of the Beijing Sport University, in particular Professor Zhang Guangde.

Participated in the international tournaments of *Dao Yin* in Beijing in 1995 and in Hang Zhou in 1997.

Awarded seventh *Duan* of *Dao Yin Yang Sheng Gong* in 2007 (Beijing Sport University).

Responsible for the teaching of *Dao Yin Yang Sheng Gong* within the Association Kunming from 1992–2009.

Teacher of *Dao Yin Yang Sheng Gong* since 2002 with the Faculty of Northern Paris UFR Health, within the framework of the University Diploma in Traditional Chinese Medicine.

Since 1998 presented two university dissertations on the use of *Dao Yin* in chronic dorso-lumbagos: a clinical study and an orthopedic study.

Presented his work to the International Congress of Chinese Medicine, the Congress of General Medicine of Medec and in other symposia.

Co-founder of the Association Kunming in 1989.

Co-founder and president of the International Institute of Dao Yin Yang Sheng Gong (IIDYYSG) since 2005.

Zhang Jian

Born on 16 September 1979 in the province of Hebei (China).

Trained in *Wu Shu* by his uncle, Professor Zhang Guangde, since 1990, then directly and daily with him in *Dao Yin Yang Sheng Gong* since 1994.

Graduate of *Wu Shu* of the Beijing Sport University in 2001.

Since 1997, has participated as a model for the videos of *Dao Yin Yang Sheng Gong* of the Beijing Sport University.

From 2005 to 2009 he assisted Professor Zhang Guangde in his teaching of the programme of the International Institute of Dao Yin Yang Sheng Gong (IIDYYSG).

Mark Atkinson

Born in 1946 in Yorkshire.

Bachelor of Education Degree from the University of Birmingham in 1969.

Thirty-year career as a schoolteacher, including 15 years as head teacher in Jersey (Channel Islands).

Practising *Tai Ji Quan* since 1980, and *Dao Yin Yang Sheng Gong* since 1993, when he met and worked with Professor Zhang Guangde in China as his first English student.

Introduced Professor Zhang and his work into the UK in 1994.

Subsequently worked with Professor Zhang and other teachers from the Beijing Sport University in China, the United States, France, Portugal and Germany.

Participated in the international tournament of *Dao Yin* in Beijing in 1995, and at that time was also granted Senior Judge status of China *Dao Yin* Association.

Created *Ru Zhi Di Zi* (outstanding and close disciple) of Professor Zhang, and his English representative in 1999.

Awarded sixth *Duan* of *Dao Yin Yang Sheng Gong* in 2006 (Beijing Sport University).

Founder and first president of the English *Dao Yin Yang Sheng Gong* Association 1999, authorised by Professor Zhang to accredit teachers of *Dao Yin Yang Sheng Gong* in England.

Founder and principal teacher of the *Dao Yin Taiji* centre in Jersey (Channel Islands) 1990–2000.

Founder and principal teacher of L'Association *Chung Fu* in Saintes, Charente Maritime, France 2001–11.

Member of the Conseil d'Administration of the International Institute of Dao Yin Yang Sheng Gong (IIDYYSG) since 2005.

Now retired and living in Norfolk.

CPI Antony Rowe
Eastbourne, UK
November 03, 2023